*a birth memoir by*

# BROOKLYN JAMES

# BORN in the

# BED you were

# MADE

One Family's Journey
from Cesarean to
Home Birth

Arena Books, Austin, Texas

Arena Books titles may be purchased for educational, business, or sales promotional use. For information, please contact:

www.brooklyn-james.com

Edited by Cynthia Gage
Cover design © Sarah Hansen, Okay Creations
Interior book design by Champagne Book Design

First Edition—December 2018
ISBN: 978-1-73081-154-8
Library of Congress Control Number: 2018913240

Printed in the United States of America
10 9 8 7 6 5 4 3 2 1

This is a work of nonfiction, and the events it recounts are true. However, certain names and identifying characteristics of some of the people who appear in its pages have been changed or excluded altogether to protect others' privacy and good name.

The perspective published in this book is in good faith. The publisher and author assume no responsibility or liability for any adverse effects from the use of information contained in this book.

# BORN in the BED you were MADE

One Family's Journey
from Cesarean to
Home Birth

# Contents

# Foreword

THERE ARE FEW TIMES IN A WOMAN'S LIFE WHERE THE PASSION OF LOVE, THE surrender of nature, and the power of the body are so evident than during the labor and birth of a child. This is her unleashing, and her complete and utter joy. The birth of a child changes everything: whether or not she realizes it, she is forever different.

There are as many different experiences of birth as there are mothers. As mothers, our stories frame who we are, who our children are, and how our children see birth. Our stories are important! They matter.

I decided after birthing four children in a hospital setting in the 1990s to become a home birth midwife. This seemed, to many, like a wild and crazy idea. When I was pregnant, I didn't know about midwives. I didn't know there was an option to birth at your home with a knowledgeable, caring woman whom you had built a relationship with during your pregnancy. I spent a total of about 45 minutes with my OB during each pregnancy. When I went into labor, I drove to the hospital, then labored in bed while connected to IV's and monitors. And when I was ready, I pushed my babies out into the hands of a doctor I hadn't even met. But I thought it was good. I wasn't induced. I hadn't had epidurals. I hadn't had any cesarean sections. My labors were fairly fast, and there were no complications. I would have been the perfect candidate for home birth. If I had only known.

After having a dream about attending a woman at her birth and a conversation about that dream with a dear friend, she invited me to her home birth. My life was changed forever. I met her midwife before the birth during a prenatal visit, and then she spent 45 minutes with her midwife at that appointment alone. The midwife addressed her fears. They talked about nutrition, her stress level, and her expectations for this birth. My friend asked questions that were answered fully, and she expressed her desires for this birth. I learned things about pregnancy and birth that I had never learned, even though I had birthed four children.

The fact of this kind of care in pregnancy was a revelation to me.

When my friend went into labor, I went to her home. We walked, we squatted, we prayed, we laughed, and we walked some more. As her labor progressed, her midwife arrived with an assistant, set up her equipment in the bedroom, monitored mama and baby intermittently between the walking, squatting, praying, and laughing, and then sat in the corner while quietly knitting.

When my friend said it was time, she climbed up on her bed, gave what I call a gentle roar, and pushed her baby out. It wasn't easy. But it was real, and it was beautiful. The energy in that room was like nothing I had ever experienced. With tears rolling down my face, I knew there was a new path for me.

I always suspected that there was more for me in birth than I had experienced. I knew that pregnancy, labor and birth held a fascination for me that I didn't quite understand. The tears at the birth of my friend's baby washed away those old expectations and assumptions. I didn't know it at that moment, but that day was the beginning of my journey to becoming a midwife.

My story is special and unique to me. I have told this story to many women and men who often ask me, how did you get into midwifery? I believe my story tells of following the path others expect of you. It tells of exploration into parts of me and of others that I never dreamed I would know. It tells of compassion and empowerment.

The story told in this book is of those same things. It shares the exquisite journey of a woman through her first pregnancy, birth by cesarean section, the loss of a pregnancy, and the ultimate surrender and trust that led to a successful vaginal home birth. It is told with the voice of a great storyteller, one who you listen to with rapt attention, cry with when her heart is breaking, and laugh out loud with as she tells you what she really thinks. Brooklyn shares her thoughts and feelings openly, asking us to listen to our own hearts and best selves who almost always know what the right answer is.

I always suggest to my clients that they write down their birth stories before time and sleep deprivation cause them to forget the details.

I was impressed and elated to read Brooklyn's thoughts and feelings about her birth experiences. I am always grateful and honored to be invited into the very intimate setting of a family's birth, and it is a great pleasure for me to invite you to read Brooklyn's birth memoir *Born in the Bed You Were Made*.

Genevieve Schaefer, LM, CPM
Sisters Midwifery, Austin, TX
July 2018

# I

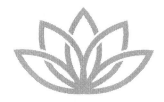

*the doing*
*was harder than*
*doing nothing*

# I Know Nothing

They're coming. Contractions. And I don't know what to do.

I should have paid attention to the title of the only pregnancy-related book I thumbed through over the past nine months. It is quite clear that *What to Expect When You're Expecting* is about...expecting.

I am no longer expecting. That cozy, magical, anticipatory stage gave way hours ago to something jarring, real, something I never anticipated.

This is not expecting. This is not pregnancy. This is labor. This is birth. I am not prepared for this.

"Don't read anything," *they* said. "It'll just scare you."

A sentiment to which I eagerly concurred.

Preeclampsia, placenta previa, nuchal cord, hemorrhage—these are but a few of the many terms that could rattle the nerves of any well-read pregnant woman. I know about these complications, as I am a registered nurse in the Postpartum Mother/Baby Unit.

I know too much. That's what got me into this predicament to begin with. I should have stayed home, gotten some rest, and gauged contraction status. Basically, I should have given labor a chance. I should not have let them induce me. But I did, because as hospital legend goes...

1. Active labor and delivery must be achieved within 12-24 hours of membrane rupture/water breaking or the following may occur:
2. increased risk of infection, which can lead to...
3. chorioamnionitis, which can lead to...
4. newborn being whisked off to NICU—Neonatal Intensive Care Unit—which is every birthing parent's worst nightmare.

Yet I know nothing. Contractions. They just keep coming. I wondered what they would feel like. Why did I stop at wondering? Why didn't I explore contractions further, at least attempt to simulate them somehow, or at best actively participate in a birthing class that may have armed me with techniques in coping with them?

For these contractions make me feel as if I am an object in a vise, a bench vise equipped with metal jaws that clamp, hold, and force something, usually wood, together in its clutches. Yes, my lower back feels like it is in that vise. I am so sorry to any piece of wood I handled in shop class, to every piece of wood I coerced into a vise that must have felt like my lumbar with every contraction. It is crushing and on the verge of splintering. The pressure is unlike anything I have ever felt. Unbearable. Unmanageable.

No longer having to wonder what contractions feel like, I am left still to wonder how will I ever get through these contractions?

I am active, upright, and pacing. It feels like the thing to do. And… oh…sweet Jesus…please…here comes another squeeze. My eyes widen like a frightened animal, nostrils flaring and snorting. My jaw—akin to my lower back—is clenched and unsupportive of oxygen flow. I lean against the sink, the wall, my husband, anything. My knees buckle under mounting pressure.

Knees. I want to get on my hands and knees. That's what instinct tells me to do. But again, I know too much. I can't get on my hands and knees on this hospital floor. Although custodial services mopped it down after the last laboring woman, it is not her germs that concern me. Oxymoronically, super-sanitized hospitals in fact have many germs and are home to "superbugs."

I can't crawl around on the floor anyhow. What am I, an animal? Yes. Yes, I am! But I would not know this until my second birth. Right now, I know nothing.

Instead of instinctively listening to my body, I aim to be logical. In the few precious minutes of rest between contractions, I squander time thinking. Think. Think. Think! Before it comes back. How am I going to get through this?

You work out, you run, you are strong. I start the pep talk to myself. You have a powerful will…right? I mean, come on, you packed up with $600 to your name and drove off in a beat-up jalopy one week after high school graduation to a city 800 miles away where you knew no one and didn't even have a place to stay, but you did...stay. You roped 200-pound calves from the saddle of a horse and wrestled them to the ground in order to tag their ears for identification purposes. You put in 16-hour days for weeks at a time in city after city with a traveling fashion show. You passed the CPAT—Candidate Physical Ability Test—for firefighters with time to spare! Heck, you survived the night shift in an Adult Medical/Surgical Intensive Care Unit straight out of a BSN program.

You're tough...right. Right? Yes!

That's how I am going to get through this. I am going to outmuscle, outrun, and outwork labor itself. That's right. I'm going to out will labor, because that's logical.

And the labor goddesses laugh.

But I don't hear them because I am too busy psyching myself up as if I am about to run the ten-mile loop at Town Lake, as if I am about to put up a one-rep max bench press. Okay, yeah, get mad at it! You got this! I'm pacing, joggling my arms and legs, limbering up...oblivious to the fact that I am wasting energy...essential energy.

Contraction. Oh...good...God. I writhe and contort, overcome with resistance and anxiety and adrenaline yet again. How am I going to get through this? This contraction has not even peaked and I am already thinking about how to get through the next one...and the next one... and the next one. The moment escapes me while my jaw seizes hold of groans and moans and roars that would give anything to escape me.

I work in this hospital. I can't make a scene. I can't growl. What am I, an animal? Yes. Yes, I am! But I would not know this until my second birth. Have I mentioned that I know nothing.

Consequently, my rational "thinking brain" repeats this fruitless cycle over and over and over again—fight, fear, flight.

The "thinking brain" is, without a doubt, impressive. This outermost, superficial, more recently evolved "new brain" used by higher mammals and humans knows a lot. The same as every other human, my new brain knows things via observation, inquiry, information, deducing. But my new brain knows nothing about birthing. Birth cannot be navigated intellectually.

Birth is best navigated by the "primitive brain." Equally impressive, this innermost, deepest "old brain" that evolved hundreds of millions of years ago giving rise to the reptilian age knows a lot, too. It is a unique kind of "knowing." Again, the same as every other human, my old brain needs no teaching; it just knows. Basic physiological functions—hormones, emotion, memory, heart rate, blood pressure, moving, resting, feeding, breathing, *birthing*—are in my old brain's wheelhouse, its primary concern to ensure my survival.[1]

Survival...

That's how I could get through this.

Reflexive, autonomic, involuntary—the old brain does without knowing it is doing. Routinely operating on the fly, reacting, and adjusting via an inherent feedback mechanism, the old brain is literally connected to the body.

I, the ego, the thinking self, I...do not know how to do this. But my body knows. My old brain knows, the brain connected to my body. The same body that has been wanting to get down on hands and knees on the floor. The same body that has been wanting to bellow, mouth open, to let go of the jaw, from the depths of its solar plexus.

That's how I could get through this.

But I don't. Unwittingly, I continue to sabotage my own efforts. I continue to listen to my new brain, which only inhibits my old brain. Mind and consciousness refuse to get out of the way, refuse to fade into the background and let intuition and body take over. I, the ego, the thinking self, I...cannot do this.

Sometime around shift change, after being up all night and enduring at least twelve hours of an artificial/induced labor, and zapped of its strength, its will, its toughness, the ego surrenders to the epidural.

Surrender...

Now there's a concept. One I wouldn't consider until left with no way out.

# Blue Curtain

Cold.

Sterile.

Blinding.

"You're so strong…and brave, babe."

"I'm so proud of you."

"I love you."

"We're really doing this."

"We're gonna meet our baby girl…any minute now."

My husband, Wade, is no longer coaching at my side in the labor room. He soothes from a chair in the operating room at the most superior position of my anatomy—my head. He is situated there for three reasons:

1. This is where his chair was placed.
2. They do not want him to see.
3. He does not want to see.

And I definitely do not want to see. I don't even want to think about what they are doing to my body, my abdomen, my uterus.

But I have seen…all the c-sections I ever want to see. Again, I know too much. That is why I am retching into a pink kidney-shaped plastic basin.

I know what they are doing behind the blue curtain. They are cutting through my skin, layer by layer, then into my fascia. Don't think about it! Retch. Get yourself together. Focus. Look at Wade. It is going to be okay. Smile.

They are separating my rectus abdominis. My abs. Abs that support my core. Abs I have grown quite fond of in my health and fitness efforts. Vain? Maybe. Nonetheless, they are separating them—abs that by nature want to contract inward and together, an intrinsic reaction to protect the organs beneath—and literally prying them apart. Don't think about it! Retch.

They have to part the abdomen to get to the peritoneum where another incision will be made exposing my guts. Yep, bowel and bladder—susceptible to nicks and damage, accidental of course. But it can and does happen. And I agreed to this? I signed off? Gave my informed consent? Don't think about it! Retch.

All of that isn't even the unnerving detail. What is unnerving is once they get my bladder pushed down and away for its own safety, they are going to cut into my uterus. My uterus which cocoons our precious baby girl—susceptible to nicks and damage, accidental of course. But it can and does happen. Retch! Retch! Retch!

I can barely feel any part of my body below the blue curtain. Just some pressure, a few tugs and pulls. C-sections are rough. There is nothing gentle about a cesarean. Cut, tug, pull, sponge, suction, cauterize, repeat. My body has to endure all of this alone because my brain has been tricked into thinking we are pain free. That is what the epidural does: blocks the transmission of pain signals to the brain by manipulating the nerve fibers that travel through the epidural space of the spinal cord. Apparently it has blocked my common sense, too. This is unnecessary, neither an emergency surgery nor a lifesaving surgery. How did it come to this? Why did you agree to this?

Don't think about it! You're okay. She's okay. Look at Wade. Focus on him. Sweet man. God, I love him. Concern and wonder whirl in his compassionate eyes, his beautiful blue eyes with an inner ring of green flecked with gold. He is such a good man. He even remembered to bring his smartphone with my labor and delivery playlist into the operating room. Dutifully, he holds it next to my ear.

If left to me and my unwillingness to jump into the smartphone pond, the playlist would have been on my gym/running MP3 player with battery life "up to eighteen hours." We just surpassed hour thirty and, quite frankly, I'm growing tired of my playlist. One more thing I failed to prepare for. Up-tempo workout songs are not that inspiring in labor. Salt-N-Pepa's *Push It* is not so cheeky after all. Guess I thought labor was going to be a party. I knew nothing.

But the song playing now doesn't bother me. It is perfect, really, a rare melancholy jam. Willie Nelson's *Blue Eyes Crying In The Rain* reminds me of my grandmother. "Gram" had blue eyes. Gram gave birth to ten of her eleven children at home. I thought about a home birth with a midwife. My insurance would not cover it. So here I am... strapped to this table. Arms straight out to the sides, think Jesus on the cross. So I do...think of him, too.

Wade, Willie, Gram, and Jesus—with the four of them present, my retching subsides.

The chatter and activity behind the blue curtain shift from routine to climactic. In an instant, relief numbs worry, as swift and direct to my system as the numbing medication through my epidural. Relief comes in the form of a vigorous wildcat cry. A wildcat cry that to this day I can hear. My eyes and Wade's eyes dart to the direction from which our just-born daughter's promising pitch comes before a swift change of course to each other's eyes. Our vision clouded amidst pooling tears, our lips seek and find connection by way of a Spiderman kiss. The room reverberates with triumphant laughter, now that we can.

"Go, babe, go," I encourage, sensing that he is conflicted. Is he supposed to stay with me or go to her?

I want to go to her. That cry does something to me. Although I am unable to feel anything below my navel, I could feel that cry. Did that lower back vise somehow latch onto my heart with its iron jaws? No. It is that cry, innocent yet formidable. It has wafted its way into my body, enveloping my heart with its needs-be-met melody.

The monitor to which the anesthesiologist has me hooked actually starts beeping, a warning sign. The little red heart flashes, lub-dubbing over one hundred beats per minute. With her hand prepped over the epidural portal in case she needs to push a larger dose of pain medication through it, the anesthesiologist asks, "Are you okay? Are you in pain?"

I shake my head. I am not in pain per se. But something is

happening. Something new and biologic—my heart, tethered to that eight-pound bundle of delectable flesh and bone that we made and has emerged from my uterus, is actually racing in response to her cry. The intrinsic reaction makes it easy for me to grasp an Elizabeth Stone quote I recently read: "Making the decision to have a child is momentous. It is to decide forever to have your heart go walking around outside your body."

I reach for her, but my arms do not cooperate. They are still tied down. All I can do is swallow the mounting lump at the back of my throat and make some sort of desperate growling sound. Her wild cry brings out something untamed in me. I want to bellow *Let me up! Give her to me!* But I don't because I know they won't. They can't. I can't. Yet it doesn't negate how much I want to be the first to hold her, be the first eyes she looks into, to smell her skin and have her smell mine, to nuzzle up together, cement that bond, claim her as my own. I carried her for thirty-nine weeks and one day already—grew her inside my womb, shared oxygen, blood, nourishment, emotions, hopes, dreams, everything—and I will carry her for the rest of my life. As soon as I can get up from this damn table.

Finally it stops…as she makes eye contact with her daddy.

"Hi, baby girl," Wade coos, mere inches in front of her face.

And she looks at him peacefully, quietly, knowingly. Yes, to him she belongs, a true born daddy's girl.

I wouldn't take that moment away from him…from them. He got to see her first. He loves that, and so does she when she recreates the story of her birth:

"…I wanted back in Mama's belly. I said 'Waaah! Waaah! Waaah!' But, but, but…then I saw Daddy. I said 'That's my daddy.' I was so happy to meet him I stopped crying…"

Wade and Mila's meeting first would be the only saving grace of that c-section.

# Nurse Curse

Has there ever been a term more misleading than "morning sickness"?

I get it. The increase of pregnancy hormones, such as progesterone and hCG—human chorionic gonadotropin—coupled with lower blood sugar levels in the morning make a fine case for morning sickness. But it only shattered expectations as I counted, day after day, the hours from morning through afternoon and deep into the night, waiting determinedly for a settled feeling in my tummy that took thirteen weeks in coming.

I never felt more like a new woman than when my "all the livelong damn day sickness" mysteriously vanished near the end of the first trimester. How can this be? I thought. I went to bed in my perpetual state of queasiness, and this morning it's gone? Just like that? Quickly coming to my senses, I stopped looking the gift horse in the mouth and instead sprinted out the door. Armed with an actual and wonderful appetite, I ordered migas and coffee. I can't say that I didn't *Oh, Yes!* my way through that meal similar to the way Meg Ryan's "Sally" climaxed through her meal in the restaurant scene in *When Harry Met Sally.*

Other than timeless nausea from week six through twelve, my medical record would show I had an "unremarkable" pregnancy, not even the slightest scare.

Despite "advanced maternal age" at thirty-five, I had never been in better shape physically or mentally. Finally comfortable in my own skin and at the pinnacle of personal health and fitness going into pregnancy, I was able to continue running and working out up until delivery.

I lost count of the number of people who approached me—in the gym, at the track, on Town Lake—when I started to show to tell me how "easy" my labor was going to be because I was "fit" and continued to exercise. So many people commented that I began to believe them, and I counted on it.

The energy was there, the ability to manage writing and music endeavors with book and music releases, and while fulfilling a steady gig schedule all while working part-time nights to keep my RN license up to scratch. However, such productivity and energy would escape me in another pregnancy. Whoever said "No two pregnancies are the same" could not have been more accurate.

In luck, my first *pregnancy* was quite effortless.

Akin to the opinions of those sweet souls—in the gym, at the track, on Town Lake—statistics would have it that if a woman is healthy going into pregnancy, and maintains that health throughout pregnancy, then labor is more likely to be healthy (i.e. shorter in duration and more effective overall). Some statistics even go so far as to say that if a woman is healthy going into labor then her requirement for pain medication is decreased.

If/then...

Remember if/then statements? Deductive reasoning? As a terrible math student, I'm not certain I do. But I think it goes something like hypothesis/conclusion. *If* two lines are perpendicular, *then* they form right angles. The tricky thing about if/then statements is that they are conditional. Still, as much as I would like it to be, it is not math's fault that my labor conclusion did not meet conditions and ultimately proved false.

Who was it that said "If you want the answer to a tough question then ask nature first"? Even Einstein...yeah, that Einstein...Albert—the dude who fundamentally changed the way we look at the universe and nature by deconstructing its inner workings—said "Look deep into nature, and then you will understand everything better."

It is quite clear to me now that interrupting nature, intervening and inducing an otherwise natural process is what put the kibosh on my labor conclusion.

But how could I have understood that? I hadn't done my homework. I hadn't questioned the highly technological medical system I was ensconced in that oft thinks its science is smarter than nature; or maybe more accurately, that does not have the patience for nature. Interrupting nature was routine, certainly not a brow-raiser, in my work environment. The majority of women I took care of in

Postpartum had some form of labor intervention. A natural medication-free, intervention-free birth in the hospital in which I worked was a rare thing.

I doubt I had the patience for nature either, my personal life easily paralleling my work life. I would have personally and eagerly supplanted "ambition" and "initiative" for "impatience" and "intervention," and thought myself a go-getter in doing so.

Impatience and intervention are a dicey duo that led to a medically unnecessary c-section in my experience. Then I finally did the natural thing...sought to justify that experience. And everyone wanted to give me a hand in finding peace of mind.

"Oh, yes, labor went on long enough. Having the c-section was the right decision," said the ob-gyn.

"I'm just thankful it's over, and that you and the baby are okay," said my mother.

"Why didn't we just do the c-section to begin with," said my husband.

"At least you aren't nursing a tear or hemorrhoids or sitting on a donut or in a sitz bath," said a coworker.

"I'm kind of jealous. I wish I could've had a c-section!" said a friend.

One of the more peculiar justifications was the *Nurse Curse*. I giggle as I admit this. Could one go so far as to validate a cesarean on a *curse*: a supernatural power to inflict harm or punishment on someone or something?

No laughing matter, the Nurse Curse is a seemingly real thing to many. Ask any nurse who has put in a little time on the floor, and I guarantee they know a nurse who has been affected by, or they have been personally affected by, or at the very least they have heard of the Nurse Curse.

The Nurse Curse has much in common with Murphy's Law: When a nurse has a medical procedure or enters a hospital as a patient, if something can go wrong...it will go wrong.

I have met many a nurse who worked in Postpartum and/or Labor & Delivery who birthed via cesarean. As it happened, a coworker whose bump stretched her scrubs to the limit, as did mine, birthed behind the blue curtain only a month or so before I did.

I distinctly remember hearing of her fate long before a c-section was even a thought, let alone an actual outcome, in my pregnancy. One of our coworkers said, "It's the nurse curse. It struck again." Little did I know that I would be the next in line for Nurse Curse remarks.

"It's that damn nurse curse, you know," said a coworker with a chuckle, attempting to keep my spirits up, as she stopped by my room in Postpartum.

"Uh-huh," I agreed with a snicker.

But did I? Agree?

If I did agree, if it was the Nurse Curse or any other rationale, if it was "failure to progress"—the most common reason for primary cesarean and of all the reasons the one most under laboring women's control—then why couldn't I shake that nagging inner voice saying, above all the celebration and smiles and justification, *what the hell happened?*

"She's okay. You're okay. That's all that matters." I must have heard the encouraging sentiment, intended to moderate irresolution, tens of times. I must have said it tens of times myself.

But was I? Okay?

That damn nag. My inner voice. Persistent bitch. Every time I would allow myself to grow comfortable in my "need" to have birthed via cesarean, she would prop herself upon my shoulder and lecture away.

You, of all people, know how important patient advocation is. You should have advocated for yourself! You should have demanded more time. You should have refused the induction altogether. How did this happen to you? You are a nurse, for crying out loud! You know most hospitals...this hospital, the one in which you work... have cesarean rates of at least thirty percent. You know your ob-gyn has a thirty percent cesarean rate. She told you so herself! One in three women will birth via cesarean. Where one in three of those women will be diagnosed with failure to progress...my ass. The World Health Organization says any cesarean rate over fifteen percent is too much, actually dangerous to maternal and newborn health.[1] Daaangerrrouuus! (She sing-sang enunciated like Oprah giving away her favorite things, before her voice slipped back into its usual low and slow burn tone.) Go ahead, lie to yourself. But you know the truth.

# Come Undone

I SUCCESSFULLY GAGGED THE NAG...FOR A WEEK, ANYWAY.

How could I focus on anything other than the beautiful creature as interested in getting to know me as I was her. Perfectly chubby. Exquisitely wobbly. The way her little body melded and molded against mine, I had to be the most familiar thing, made explicitly for her.

Softness, fragility, vulnerability—characteristics I grew up fighting, overcoming, surely never admiring—on her were flawless. So appealing I had neither the desire nor the fortitude to resist them. Yes, in her presence, I was as soft, as fragile, as vulnerable as she.

Yet I was a rock. As was she. Intrinsically born with trust and expectation, she was determined I would and could provide. Following her cues, sometimes as subtle as a smacking of the lips, other times as palpable as her signature wildcat cry, I was equally determined to provide. That immediate trust and expectation gave me the confidence to do so.

She had these slate gray eyes, commanding yet seeking and nearly impossible to look away from, intensely curious and wise beyond her knowing.

"Babies make you believe in God because there's something just beyond understanding about their freshness and fragility and their smell and their toes. When they take their first breaths, and when they land, floppy and slippery, on your chest...when you watch their tiny sleeping selves, when you hear their thin wild animal cries, you know, you just know in your guts that God is real, and that babies have been with him more recently, have come more directly from him than our worn-out old selves have." —Shauna Niequist

Yes, this child, my child, our child had been with God. She knew things we didn't, a messenger maybe. And I saw...in those slate gray eyes...the mother, the woman, the person I want to be. A child, a changer of lives, a vessel through which transformation and understanding flow, and here I thought we would be the teachers.

Those unparalleled moments of newborn sweetness, coupled with the learning curve that defines "rookie parent," kept that nag off my shoulder. Maybe she was there, yacking away as usual, but I was too busy or too tired to hear. More so, I was too grateful to question.

Seven nights after being cut open and stitched back up, that gratitude began its shift from modern medicine to a primordial body—an instinctive body, a body operating on autopilot at the control of the "old brain"—my primordial body that knew enough to unstitch itself.

This physical unraveling would be the catalyst to a spiritual unraveling of what type of labor and birth I truly wished I had, of what type of labor and birth I would long for and prepare myself for in the future, of what type of labor and birth for which I would personally form a strong conviction.

On the whole, I avoid the word "conviction" because it brings to mind a sentencing or, even worse, politics. But we all have convictions—ideas, opinions, beliefs. One of the more effective, or maybe more appreciated, beliefs being objectivity: "To each their own."

I am not anti-cesarean.

A testament to what a birthing body is willing and capable of withstanding to bring forth life, cesarean birth is nothing if not extraordinary. The only option for some, cesareans and ob-gyns/surgeons who perform them can and do save lives, nothing short of miraculous. A choice for others, cesareans can and do provide desired outcomes/exemplary births.

I do not dispute medically necessary cesarean birth. I know no one who does.

Even elective cesarean, for breech position or following primary cesarean or because that is simply the type of birth a woman chooses for herself or for any other reason, is no more for me to debate than my home birth is for someone else to scrutinize.

I generally believe every woman should be encouraged to labor and deliver as she so desires, be that with or without pain-relieving medication, vaginally, cesarean, in a hospital, at home, in a tub, on a bed, or on the moon! Whereas, I personally believe every woman should be encouraged to give herself the chance to birth as naturally, humanistically, transformatively as possible.

But I did not know that…initially. Remember, I knew nothing. I would not know I had any convictions about birth until I did not get the birth I wanted. As Randy Pausch said, "Experience is what you get when you didn't get what you wanted."

Unfortunately, you can't tell me anything. Sure, you can try, but I am one of those overly optimistic, bold, naïve, bordering on foolish leapers who has to experience it to get it, who must jump in and sink before anything sinks in.

No, I didn't know how I wanted to birth in my first pregnancy. Until a woman is pregnant, how much does she know about being pregnant? And until a woman is in labor, how much does she know about laboring? Let alone how she wants to labor.

I did ask a few friends and family members about their experiences. By "experiences," I alluded to their labors and births, giving nary a thought to how they *prepared* for those labors and births, which I would later discover made all the difference.

Those experiences run the gamut. With as varying ways to birth as there are to order coffee at Starbucks—vaginal, a little tear is fine, no episiotomy, please; let me try a non-cesarean, pain-free, extra shot of epidural; induction with a side of mechanical extraction, vaccum, no forceps, please; I'll take a repeat cesarean, as it comes; straight-up, fully charged spontaneous birth, hold the meds and interventions, please— most compared contractions to pain they had never felt before and two actually described them as uncomfortable but "not painful." Of course I ran with the latter, believing my contractions could be only uncomfortable, too! Most were hospital births with the exception of one birthing center birth, and an aunt who attested that she had her children "everywhere" as she routinely experienced "precipitous labor" where she birthed quite rapidly, and unplanned, a few children at home, a few children in the car on the way to the hospital, and a few children in next to no time upon reaching the hospital.

If I wanted to know about planned home birth, I would've had to have asked Gram, the coolest lady I ever knew who had ten of her eleven children at home. Not because it was en vogue or the latest birth trend, but out of necessity for rural working-class women in the 1920s and 1930s. But Gram was gone. After ninety-two years on this earth, she had been gone nearly twenty. And gone with her was a slew of knowledge. Not "book smarts" or anything one learns in medical school. Just common sense, seasoned *been there, done that* invaluable resourcefulness. It's a shame, especially when it comes to something so sacred as birth—a rite of passage—that we seem to have abandoned the tradition of inherited knowledge in exchange for science and convenience.

"Home birth" was merely a term to me, an elusive notion. In retrospect, I believe it was more a subconscious desire. Upon finding out we were pregnant, I called my health insurance provider to inquire if they would cover a home birth. Any intent, and instinct, to seek a midwife under whose care I could birth at home was prematurely squashed when I discovered that my insurance did not support and would not cover home birth.

I had neither witnessed a planned home birth nor personally knew anyone who had. Taking birth out of the home and into the hospital took away firsthand learning for young women. What I knew about birth prior to nursing school was what I saw on television and in movies. Ugh. What I knew about birth after nursing school was based on my experience working in a hospital. Double ugh. The first birth I ever saw at twenty-two years old was in a hospital. No news flash. It was an artificially induced labor resulting in an episiotomy/vacuum-assisted delivery. I was stunned, stupefied. *What the hell happened?*

It was 1999, ergo I stood, pay phone in hand, unable even to form words to describe my older sister's birth to our eldest sister.

"Sis, you there?" she asked, again.

"Uh-huh," I finally mumbled.

"So, did she have the baby?"

"Uh-huh."

"Is she okay?"

"Uh-huh."

"Is the baby okay?"

"Uh-huh."

"Are you okay?"

"Unh-uh."

It was traumatic. Episiotomies, controversial in causing more harm than they prevent,[1] are gruesome. Blood. All I remember is blood…and a lot of it. In hindsight, rather than highlighting STDs in rudimentary Sex Ed classes, they may as well show a *typical* hospital birth if they really want to scare our youth into abstinence.

My sister was okay. My beautiful bouncing niece, the first of a new generation, was okay. But they could have been a lot better if not for the episiotomy and vacuum. My niece developed a cephalohematoma, which is pooling of blood and bruising on the skull from the vacuum. And, good God, that episiotomy had to hurt, both in receiving and healing. My sister did it all without an epidural, without any pain-relieving medication whatsoever. She may as well have birthed at home! Saved herself the episiotomy and saved our niece the cephalohematoma.

Experiences leave impressions, be they conscious or dormant. They are stored in the brain, the body, the soul, somewhere, maybe everywhere. It is unfortunate yet quite logical that the perplexity of my first birth matched that of the first birth I ever witnessed. *What the hell happened?*

A little more than a term, an elusive notion, I took the time to make a "birth plan." Something coworkers told me not to do: "The surest way to screw up your birth is to make a plan and write it down." That hunch, as the Nurse Curse, is not solely based in superstition but in materialization. I cannot recall any woman I took care of in Postpartum who had a formalized birth plan in her chart whose plan did not get derailed at some point during the birthing process. Or, could it be, little to do with the birth plan or the Nurse Curse, the common thread being the hospital?

Even my birth plan lacked conviction. I didn't want to be induced. But if I had to be induced, I preferred to start with Cervidil versus going straight to Pitocin. I wanted to birth without pain medication for as long as I could, but I wasn't opposed to an epidural if I needed one. I wanted as much privacy as possible. However, if a resident or student nurse was on the floor and needed the experience, they could come in. After all, I was once in their shoes.

The only hard lines on my birth plan were no cesarean, no episiotomy, and no vacuum. The last two absolutes obviously stemmed from the memory of my sister's birth. Although I didn't have a clear vision of what my birth would look like, I knew what it wouldn't look like. It would not involve major surgery.

Alas...

Major surgery I had. And it all—surgery, blind faith in the medical birth model, birth ambivalence—was about to come undone.

# Standing Orders

MY MOTHER DID NOT BREASTFEED ME. UNTIL MY POSTPARTUM NURSING STINT and subsequent pregnancy, I never gave it a thought. Did I miss out on something? Did my immune system miss out on something? The digestive tract, where bacteria and the immune system meet, is the cornerstone of the immune system with up to eighty percent of immune tissue residing there. Breastfeeding has been shown to positively affect immune system health and long-term health in not only infants and toddlers but in mothers, too. Did my mother also miss out on something?

Mom birthed and parented in an era when formula and its supplements—canned/evaporated milk, Karo syrup, and rice cereal—had surpassed breastfeeding in promising a more effective, precise, and affordable way to feed babies. I reckon she never gave it a thought either. Whether due to generational or socioeconomic factors or individual choice, informed or not, Mom, who was breastfed herself to some extent, said "I wanted nothing to do with it."

Interestingly enough, when Mom is around and I breastfeed, she hovers. A smile and a look of wonder at the giving and receiving, the sweetness...at what she missed?

I could have missed it, too. The same as I hadn't witnessed much natural labor and birth, I hadn't witnessed much natural nourishment either. Clearly, I had seen more cleavage on magazine covers and on women going about their ordinary days than I had on anyone breastfeeding.

If not for the hospital in which I worked, I would have remained uninformed and unexposed. It was in this hospital where I found myself captivated by breastfeeding art that adorned the walls of the Postpartum wing. It was in this Postpartum wing where I witnessed nurses and lactation consultants who respected and provided resources for any woman who did not desire to breastfeed equally encourage and educate any woman who had the desire to breastfeed. Amazing! Beautiful! Empowering! I thought. Women breastfeed? Yes, they do! Not only educational but inspiring, an instance where hospital policy provided resources for and propped up individual choice.

I had learned so much from this hospital. I had grown to adore the staff who took me under their wings and showed me the ropes in my novice position.

Why, then, was I in such a hurry to get out…as a patient?

I spent more hours in the hospital laboring and birthing than I did in postpartum recovery. It was so strange. As if the removal of the epidural after surgery not only allowed feeling to return to my body but allowed feeling to return to my will.

You're going to take issue now? After the fact? I couldn't help but question myself, or my will.

I knew well the daily and nightly grind on Postpartum. The "standing orders" in my chart would state that for twenty-four hours post-cesarean, I should remain on Pitocin and IV fluids. The IV in my hand should stay in place. The urinary catheter, inserted along with the epidural, should remain in place until the effects of the epidural wore off and I could safely ambulate to and from the bathroom and effectively relieve my bladder of its urine, epidurals sometimes complicating this otherwise reflexive process. I should sit up on the edge of the bed, stand if I felt I could, within the first twelve hours postoperatively, yada yada yada.

Standing orders, "ensuring continuity of procedure" irrespective of individuality, similar to standardized tests, can sometimes be unreliable. I knew the orders could be changed if a patient asks. Question being, do most patients know they can ask?

We transferred to Postpartum around two-thirty in the morning. After catching a few z's, and after the on-call doctor rounded early that same morning, I put in my order to have everything removed…yesterday. No more IV, no more Pitocin or fluids, no more catheter, nothing. I wanted to be intervened upon no more.

And I wanted to be discharged…the day before yesterday. I felt fine.

I wasn't having much pain, considering what my body had been put through at my consent. I was mobile, with the exception of dragging around one leg which persisted in its numbness hours after discontinuing an overall one-sided epidural. Although I was happy to drag it around versus lie in that bed any longer.

Maybe this need to get up was my rally cry, my way of making everything okay—march on, don't look back, focus on what's ahead and important. Baby girl was finally with us. Leary of and dead set against any separation from or intervening upon her, I wanted and needed to take her home. And they let us the next morning, as early as I could round up a doctor to sign off on our discharge papers.

While most hospitals pride themselves on striving for continuity of care—an idealized patient experience by being provided high-quality care with an identified healthcare provider—I had seen how that does not always happen. And in my personal inpatient experience, I saw how frustrating that can be. I couldn't identify any of the rounding doctors I saw in Postpartum, and I worked there, albeit part-time. One might have thought it was Christmas; to be fair, it was five days before.

All of that rallying—getting up—for naught. Even in leaving, they insisted I sit back down. Hospital policy, all postpartum women must be escorted from their rooms to their vehicles via wheelchair regardless of ability and/or desire to walk. And I have been a part of this...enforced the policy and personally wheeled mothers, perfectly capable and wanting to walk, out of the hospital? Yes? Yes, I have.

Once the wheels hit the welcome mat just outside the automatic sliding doors, *Clink! Clink!* went the footrests, my toes slapping them up against the leg rests, with the wheelchair and hospital policy coming to an abrupt halt.

"Thank you," I said to the LVN guiding the wheelchair as I bounded out, never so impatient to stand on my own two feet. See! You're fine! She's fine! My nagging inner voice unleashed herself, challenging the doctors, the hospital, and their procedures. She's standing! Ha ha ha haaa! Put that in your standing orders pipe and smoke it!

Oh, shut up, I beseeched whatever part of my subconscious she represented. I knew she was a hothead, but an ignoramus, too? Surely she had butchered that idiom.

I hugged the LVN. I knew her, had worked with her. She is a lovely lady who didn't write the hospital policy, and probably didn't always agree with it, but she had to do her job. Then I bounded into the truck.

"Easy, babe," Wade said, his chivalrous yet empty hand still awaiting mine as he closed me in the backseat alongside baby girl in her car seat.

A moment forever frozen in time…

At thirty-five years of age and newlyweds, it was a moment that seemed both a lifetime and a flash in coming. We had been expecting as long as we had been married. We had each grown accustomed to our own carefree lifestyles, and carried that free and easy vibe into the lifestyle we were building as man and wife. Yes, we had come and gone as we pleased longer than we had childhood curfews. Anything other was bound to be a shock to the system.

A moment that put into perspective the fact that no matter how we processed our thirty-hour birth, it was a spit in the sea of what lay ahead. We entered the hospital expecting. We left the hospital expected to parent a child.

Once settled in the driver's seat, Wade looked at me through the rearview mirror. Our eyes locked, neither smiling nor frowning, somewhere between fear and joy. The symbolism was perfect: life as we had known it was in that rearview mirror.

# Katie Holmes' Smile

A WEEK AFTER MY "FAILURE TO PROGRESS" AND SUBSEQUENT CESAREAN, A TRUE failure to listen to instinct, yet again, would no longer be denied. I, and my cesarean, came undone.

We were at my mother-in-law's annual Christmas dinner and gift exchange. Such a pleasurable tradition; she goes all out for Christmas. Somewhere between the prime rib and Yorkshire pudding, I could not tolerate another bite. If only it were because I ate too much.

My abdomen was so sore. It had been giving me fits for the past couple of days. Its tenderness made even walking painful, yet I kept walking because I knew how important that was postoperatively. It was huge, seemingly larger than when I was pregnant. And it was bruising... from my navel to my thighs.

Are you really even a nurse? Any sensible person might wonder. Sure, I knew it was not normal.

But I wanted it to be.

I needed it to be.

I had a newborn to take care of. A newborn who breastfed every hour and a half to three hours...24/7. My milk had come in. We made it through a few days of engorgement, starting to establish some ebb and flow in our supply and demand. We did not need any setbacks. I barely had time to sleep, let alone to sit in a doctor's office, or, God forbid, an emergency room. Whatever was wrong with my abdomen/ insides would have to fix itself. And it basically did.

I caved and called my ob-gyn's office the morning of Christmas Eve, five days postpartum, because I knew this is what any "prudent" nurse would do. I didn't want them to tell me I needed to come in, but if they had I would have. I wanted them to tell me this was fine, everything was okay, these things happen sometimes, and it will pass. Lucky for me, that's what she—the nurse practitioner, to be exact—said.

"Well...I'm concerned because I'm starting to bruise from my navel to my thighs. Mostly purple in color, some starting to yellow," I emphasized this part, knowing old bruising turns yellow. Could I convince the NP, as well as myself, whatever happened was already healing as evidenced by the yellowish-brown areas?

"Maybe a collection of blood?" My voice had an upward inflection, having enough medical experience to identify hematoma signs, before skirting around my own question. "Or maybe they just got a little rough in the section." No upward inflection needed, no question about it, cesareans are rough. "And the incision looks fine. No redness, no heat, no swelling. I don't have a fever. Just the bruising, is all."

"Well…some bruising is normal," the NP fed right into my minimizing. After all, who wants to see an unscheduled patient the morning of Christmas Eve when the office closes at noon? "What's your pain level?"

"Nothing compared to labor!" I chortled. "Just a constant dull nagging ache. I've been alternating ice and heat, and compressing it with a postpartum belly binder. That seems to ease the pain."

"I can call in another prescription of Norco?" her voice took over the upward inflection role. Norco—a mix of acetaminophen and hydrocodone—is a controlled substance, with a high risk for addiction and dependence, used to treat pain.

"No, that's okay." I had plenty left from the prescription they sent home with me postoperatively.

And, oh, the irony. It didn't hit me then, only now in hindsight. But that's what history does, doesn't it.

For PROM—"premature rupture of membranes" before onset of active labor—I was prescribed Cervidil followed by Pitocin, both medications, drugs. Those drugs required more drugs infused via an epidural to sustain. That "cascade of intervention," cascade of medication, ultimately led to a cesarean, requiring more and more and more drugs. Medication, drugs that healed nothing, treated nothing, solved nothing, only caused everything.

There I was, calling in with bruising from my navel to my thighs, possibly a hematoma, and I was offered more medication, drugs. "Pain pills" that are not going to heal, treat or solve a possible hematoma. All without even seeing me, without even saying "Why don't you come in, we'll have a look and go from there."

She didn't say it, so I felt compelled to say, "I mean, I know it's Christmas Eve, but maybe I should come in?"

"I really don't think you need to. I think it's fine. Like I said, some bruising is completely normal," the NP reiterated. Aha!...music to my ears.

"Okay, great. I'll just keep an eye on it then." And stay home with baby girl!

"Yes, do. And if you feel it's getting worse, don't hesitate to call." Easy for her to say, as she would not be the one to answer. The answering service would, taking over at noon until the morning after Christmas, referring anyone with imminent concern to the nearest emergency room.

"Will do. Well...Merry Christmas!"

"Merry Christmas to you, too."

We both got what we wanted, really. She did not want to deal with me, the unscheduled patient two hours before closing on Christmas Eve, and I did not want to be dealt with.

Consequently...

There I was salivating, eager to enjoy the rare treat of Yorkshire pudding. But my abdomen would not allow it. The pressure just kept building. It didn't feel like gas. It didn't feel like cramps. It felt like a brick. Like someone had hit me as hard as they could in the breadbasket with a Louisville Slugger.

And that "fine" incision I bragged about to the NP was starting to act up. It was hurting...in the top right-hand corner where a marble-sized hard knot formed that was tender to the touch. Not only tender but taut, the scar drew up on that side, the "bikini cut" far from the inconspicuous, straight, horizontal line I was promised.

I sneaked into the bathroom, more like waddled, still wearing pregnancy pants because my bruised and swollen belly required them. Upon pulling up my long-waisted sweater and pulling down my high-waisted pants, there in the mirror looking back at me was Katie Holmes' smile. Yes, that is what…who…my now asymmetrical surgical scar reminded me of. Although I must admit I did not find the scar as cute, in any fashion, as the famous and signature half grin.

"Motherfucker," I muttered under my breath.

Not very Christmassy. Not very new mom-ish. But very sincere. Pain and disappointment bring out the sailor mouth in me.

And I heard James Lipton from *Inside the Actors Studio* asking me question number seven of his famous series of ten: What is your favorite curse word?

Maybe it is because the f-word was forbidden in my mother's house. Forget washing one's mouth out with soap. So much as thinking about saying the f-word may have been grounds for being forced to eat the whole bar. Maybe it is because I never said the f-word until I was in my early thirties. Honestly. I thought about saying it…a bunch of times. But for my mother, I abstained. That is until one time while changing out spark plugs, I broke one off in the engine. Anyone who has ever broken off a spark plug in an engine knows it as a curse-worthy offense. It finally slipped…and, oh, the liberation!

It was so liberating in this instance that I exited the bathroom at least pretending to be in the holiday spirit, no one the wiser. After all, with dinner finished, there were presents to open.

# Open

LATER THAT EVENING WE HAULED IN OUR CHRISTMAS SCORE, MOCKING HOW exceptionally good we were for Santa to have been so generous, while the most exceptionally good thing we ever did fell asleep in her car seat on the ride home.

It had to be ten-thirty by the time we got settled in. Why does everything hurt worse at night? Recollections of ear infections and tonsillitis as a kid, it always hurt worse just in time for bed. Twenty-some-odd years shy of being a kid, nothing much has changed. I hurt.

Wade caught me in the kitchen, in passing. That is how we hugged these days...in passing, baby girl rightly taking up the majority of our time. I had come from breastfeeding her, and Wade was headed to change and swaddle her for bed.

"You alright, Mama?" he asked, taking pleasure in trying out our new titles.

"Just tired of hurting, Daddy." I hugged him tightly to me. He always feels so good to hug. Although a double-edged sword in this instance, the hug allowed me to siphon his strength but the sheer tenderness of it preyed upon my tears.

"Let's get my girls to bed," he said.

On the way to brush my teeth, I got sidetracked helping him with kick-ass swaddle technique, a skill I picked up from kick-ass preceptor nurses in Postpartum. I may have the technique, but he has the touch. In our teamwork, my hands methodically spread out and fold over and press one corner of the muslin blanket while his hands seamlessly cradle and glide and align baby girl's shoulders with the fold. My efficiency getting its moment to shine, she is swaddled like an itty-bitty burrito in seconds.

Although the swaddle is calming, her sleepy slate gray eyes refuse to close, too curious about the animated faces perched above. Her bowed mouth stays parted and on ready, if only she could get the words out. The rounded softness of her newborn cheek begs of my lips. As I bend to kiss her, a gush of something warm and wet floods from my abdomen and down the front of my pants.

Dark red blood. It appears to be a fair amount. But akin to spit-up, it is never as much as it seems. Dark red blood—old blood. Wonder how long it has been in there? Blood is a breeding ground for bacteria. I don't feel funny. I don't have a temp. It's dark, so chances are I am not actively bleeding anymore.

The drawn-up part of my incision, where the marble-sized knot formed above, has dehisced—come open—about half an inch. In addition to what ran down the front of my pants, I have collected a sanitary pad full of old dark red blood. Sanitary pads are not just for vaginas, apparently. I have worn them, as instructed, over my incision postoperatively to keep it clean and dry. Little did I know, when I gave my informed consent for cesarean, I would change them out over my incision for the same reason I change them out under my vagina!

I hurl/spike/slam the saturated pad into the garbage can. I want to curse again, but I don't. Repetition takes away the punch.

Why is this happening? My cesarean is literally coming apart at the seams? A believer in the idea that sometimes good things must fall apart in order for better things to fall together, I can't catch a glimpse of the "better" in this.

Manhandling another pad from its outer wrap, I slap it against the winking and weeping and warped incision, simultaneously mashing on the marble-sized knot above. The pad slowly fills with old dark red blood. After repeating this campground first aid a few times over, I wonder how much blood could hoard itself in my abdominal cavity without causing serious damage. It is never as much as it seems, I remind myself. And the release of blood actually flattens the knot and relieves the stinging pain with it.

Not the usual one but two "nags" duke it out on my shoulders.

You should at least call someone, tell them what's going on.

No, don't call anyone! That's what got you into this mess to begin with!

And we're back to that?

We never left that!

She had to call her doctor when her water broke.

Her water didn't break; it dribbled! And she should've stayed her ass home, got some rest, just like she should now!

She should call someone, her doctor, a doctor, any doctor.

She did! Two days ago! And they told her it was "normal"!

Well, she should call again.

She should listen to her body!

First, I listened to the nag who doesn't yell everything. I called my ob-gyn's office and got the answering service, of course. As predicted and per protocol, they referred me to the nearest ER. That is when the screamer got her way. I told the answering service that it was highly unlikely I would go to the ER and to please let my ob-gyn know what was going on, that I would be in her office first thing tomorrow morning.

It felt strange not going to the ER or urgent care or somewhere. I was a nurse, for crying out loud. If I were manning a nurse telephone triage line and someone called in to report they were bleeding from a dehisced surgical incision, wouldn't I tell them to go to the nearest emergency room or at least urgent care?

Isn't that what we do? Responsively in Western culture? Something's wrong, fix it, intervene…immediately. Why? Because we can. We have all the technology, all the conveniences.

I wanted none of it, neither technology nor convenience. At the time I chalked it up to being tired. But it was more than that. Something was brewing within me. Subtle, maybe even subliminal, I was not fully conscious of the fact that my "new brain"—the "thinking brain"—was beginning to align with my body, the knowing body fueled by the "old brain" where instinct and intuition rule. Apparently, it and I did not stomach well being cut open.

A first of many tests, how could my thinking brain and knowing body best work together? Could my thinking brain shut up long enough to listen to my knowing body? Could my intellect acknowledge the wisdom of my instinct, integrating with it rather than feeding its own ego?

What to do?

I felt fine. Innately, I knew this could wait until morning. It had been a week already. It could wait until morning, and I could save myself the exorbitant cost of emergency care. There was no need to drag baby girl out to the ER so she wouldn't miss a breastfeeding. There was no need to lose sleep. There was no need to disrupt anything...the way my labor was disrupted, the subconscious thought had to be driving this decision.

Yes, stay put.

I kept a pad tucked into the waistband of my underwear to sop up any blood that was still draining in an effort to keep the incision clean and dry. With every breastfeeding throughout the night, I took my temperature, eyeballed the incision, changed out pads, hydrated, and looked inside my body for signs and symptoms of distress.

It is amazing, in retrospect, how easily one can give up independence to the medical system without even questioning dependence. How easily I...thirty hours amidst a hard-fought labor...gave up my independence, depending on a medical system that ultimately gave me a medically unnecessary cesarean. Sure, there are true emergency and nonemergency cases that warrant our Western culture's superlative medical care. A care for which I, and countless others, am grateful. I do not dispute that.

Equally indisputable is the reality that our bodies are often smarter, maybe more in tune is the appropriate summation, than we are. For the past week my body had been working, unbeknownst to me, to fix this hematoma. To fix this hematoma caused by man, by surgery. This hematoma that could have easily required re-hospitalization, repeat surgery, even blood transfusion in the worst-case scenario.

Thankfully and with no kudos of my own, I escaped that on account of my body "treating" itself. Before I, in my thinking brain, realized anything was askew, my knowing body was already working, correcting, managing. After it became evident, and in the face of my thinking brain's denial and hope that bruising from my navel to my thighs was normal, my body steadily trudged on beneath the surface—fixing, repairing, absorbing. Still after ob-gyn diagnosis and treatment, when all was said and done, it would be up to my body to right this surgical wrong.

If my body could do this, fix a mess it didn't even make, couldn't it have done something it was expressly and biologically made to do—deliver a baby without being cut open?

That is what cesarean did for me: Opening my body, my uterus, was the catalyst to opening my eyes. And I was only beginning to see.

# Dumb Luck

"How are you even walking?" my ob-gyn asks. The look on her face matches the tone of her voice—dismay—assessing my hot-air-balloon abdomen and puckered cesarean incision. "You look like you've been in a car wreck," she continues. "Seriously, doesn't it hurt?"

"Hell, yes, it hurts." My colorful belly jiggles like St. Nick's, a nervous chuckle waning. Her reaction makes me second-guess my decision not to go to the ER. I can tell this is not something she deals with on a regular basis.

"Why didn't you call…earlier?" She can tell by the yellowish-brown areas that the bruising did not appear overnight.

"I did." My nervous chuckle waxes to the acrimonious.

"You called? With this?" The palms of her hands circle above my abdomen and incision. "When? And who did you talk to…specifically?"

"Yes. The day before Christmas. I talked with your NP. But it was right before you closed for the holiday." Was I making excuses for the NP or myself?

"And you told her about this?" Again, the palms of her hands sweep above the varicolored skin of my core.

"Yes. I told her I had bruising from my navel to my thighs." My "navel" and "thighs," like her "this," accentuated by my hands in pointing out the bruised areas.

"And you didn't come in? She didn't tell you to come in?"

"She said some bruising is normal."

"I'll be right back."

"I didn't really want to come in anyway," I call after her hasty exit.

"Ba-a-abe…" Wade expires from his seat next to the examination table upon which I lie. "We should've come in. You're the nurse, why didn't you tell me how serious this was?" His question, meant neither to be answered nor to point the finger, stems from love and concern.

"Wonder how baby girl's doing?" My reciprocal question, not

meant to be answered either, is a simple rebuttal. The first time we have been without her since she was born is as strange as I thought it would be. We should not be here. We should be with her.

Besides, Wade must be wondering if this is going to become a routine thing—me on an exam table with him seated in the vicinity. First with the c-section and now with a postpartum checkup that is five weeks early in coming.

"I want you to look at something," my ob-gyn's parental tone carries down the hallway as she nears the door to our room. In she comes, the NP follows. "This…" again with the palms of her hands "…is not normal." She looks at the NP expectantly, who looks at me almost as expectantly. "This is a hematoma. When someone calls with this much bruising…" and again with the palms of her hands "…we need to see them…immediately." The NP nods, much like the scolded child she must identify with in this moment. "Just so we're clear…this is not normal." And, yes, again with the palms of her hands.

"Okay." I give mediation an attempt and go ahead and throw myself under the bus along with the NP, "I'm sure I could've been more convincing. And now that we know it's not normal, what exactly caused it?" I pause before finding the courage to ask the question that has been hounding me, "Did I cause it?" A habitual self-pusher, always thinking I can do more…I did do more. "Did I do too much too soon?"

The answer, a relief to my conscience, only in the long run made me question the conscience of the medical model of birth.

I developed a surgically induced hematoma from an actively bleeding blood vessel that was either cauterized unsuccessfully or not at all. The blood, having no other place to go but into surrounding tissue where it is obviously not supposed to be, caused an inflammatory response as the body attempts to repair itself, resulting in pain, swelling, and bruising. The larger the bleed, the larger the hematoma. A doozy had I.

"They missed something," my ob-gyn says plain and simple, her expression a mixture of humble pie and apology.

"They missed something?" Wade speaks up, appalled at this reality.

All he knows of doctors is what many of us know of doctors: they are supposed to be gods. Capable of great feats, saving lives, they are supposed to be extraordinarily perfect, especially when taking care of our loved ones. They can't possibly be human like the rest of us, capable of making mistakes.

"How often do they 'miss something?' I mean, how often does 'this' happen?" I ask, unable to keep my tone from growing indignant. Get it together, I coach myself, uncertain if I want to cry or to give a tongue-lashing, far too easy to forget one's own imperfections when focused on another's.

"Not often," my ob-gyn answers.

Ah, yeah, that won't do. That is not at all the answer I want. I proceed, seemingly confused that I sit on the exam table of an ob-gyn and not on the couch of a psychologist. "I don't want to come off as disrespectful, but I have to tell you, I am having a hard time with all of this. First the c-section, now this. I don't have time for this. I have a newborn to take care of. It's just been so disappointing, unfulfilling. It was my first birth. I mean, it didn't have to be perfect. But, come on. It's just not in any way what I might have imagined."

"Well…" I could see her making a conscious effort to say something in which I could find comfort. "If it makes you feel any better, most births do not go exactly as planned."

Hmm…did that…make me feel better? "How many exactly turn out like mine? With a post-cesarean hematoma?"

"I'd be hard-pressed to give you a statistic. Really, I'd have no idea." She shrugs, thinking and wanting to give me something. "Maybe one percent? It is very rare."

For a guesstimate, she was quite accurate, that post-cesarean hematoma/packing/dehiscence occur in one to one and a half percent of cases.[1]

"Rare? But it happened to me." The words—embarrassing and maybe even ungrateful—flow from my mouth as I try to process how something that only happens in one percent of cesareans happened to me.

She nodded her head with understanding before sharing with me her personal birth stories, one very touch and go, far beyond anything I am experiencing now. I really like her. Her bedside manner is good, caring and conversational. She is trying to help me here. She is listening to me, sympathizing with me, even sharing her own birth stories, which did not go exactly as she had planned either.

Sitting on her exam table, I know there are people in this life who would give anything for their only medical/health problem to be a post-cesarean hematoma. I know that to some, I must sound ungracious. I even scolded myself multiple times over the past week. Stop. Just stop. There are people who have real health issues. There are babies born who go straight to NICU. Babies. You've seen them. Some of them have to fight the rest of their lives just to live and breathe and be. And you're bitching about a cesarean? About the side effects of a cesarean? Just be grateful. Baby girl is here and healthy. That is all that matters.

But apparently that was not all. I could not let it go. Something inside me kept asking, kept questioning, "Would you have recommended the same thing? If you had been there? Would we have gone to section?"

"Oh, yes," she did not hesitate. "You gave it a great effort. So did the on-call doc, giving you some leeway over the twenty-four hour mark in the event of your water breaking prematurely. I mean, you know the risk of infection that it carries. The section was the best, safest decision at that point."

Safest? I keep the challenging thought to myself. Instead I ask a hypothetical question, reaching for reason in the chain of events, attempting although very ineffectively to make sense of them somehow. "Would this have happened if you had been there to perform the section?"

"I can't say." She shrugs, understandably thrown by such a question. "I mean, there are obvious risks. That's why patients must review and consent for c-sections. But what I can say is that it can happen to anyone." She shrugs again. "It is very rare, though."

Stop saying that! I get it. Like a bloody steak, it is rare. But every time you say that it makes me think I, or the on-call ob-gyn, am defective in some way. Why did it happen to us? I try to suppress the thankless thoughts, with no luck. The nucleus of my consternation still unresolved, the cringeworthy statement finds its way out of my mouth once more: "But it happened to me."

When I signed the consent form I knew there was a laundry list of possible complications. I just never imagined any of them would apply to me. It was as if I viewed my signature as a mere technicality rather than an actual acceptance of responsibility of all the things that could go wrong. The on-call ob-gyn, genuinely wanting to provide me with comfort, only added to my blasé attitude about the risks with his reassurances that "I do this all the time. Surgery is my specialty. You'll be in and out in thirty minutes."

Even when, in all my vanity, I asked how he was with a scalpel, further getting to my point of how the scar would look, he gave me the A-OK gesture—his thumb and index finger making a circle—and said, "You won't even see it."

To which shoulder nag who yells everything, with a little Monday morning quarterbacking and a hand gesture of her own, rebukes *Tell that to Katie Holmes' smile!*

But on this Friday morning, my ob-gyn surely is growing tired of the overlong therapy session. She must be even further behind schedule than usual, what with my unscheduled appointment. She has followed triage protocol to a tee in seeing me first. She has shown compassion in spending extra time with me. I seek an answer for which there is not one definitively. What more can she say?

She shrugs again and says, "Dumb luck."

Yep. Dumb luck. Last I knew dumb luck is when something *good* happens by chance. But now is not the time for an etymology lesson. Now seems to be the time for James Lipton's question number seven, which begs of me to answer it. Shoulder nag who yells everything goes one step further, I double-dog dare you! Say it! Then shoulder nag who doesn't yell everything, who sounds a whole lot like my mother, by the way, gasps at both of us, You can't say that, especially not in a doctor's office.

I settle on, "Well…son of a bitch," simmering irritability masked in a cool and dry delivery.

Although I could not appreciate the last-ditch answer, my ob-gyn was right.

Without the complication of the hematoma, I don't believe I would have questioned the cesarean as much. It would not have felt so wrong, so unsafe, so left to chance, speaking of luck. I probably would have scheduled a repeat cesarean for our second birth because that is often what is recommended by ob-gyns. Even though, the American Congress of Obstetricians and Gynecologists recognizes vaginal birth after cesarean—commonly referred to as VBAC—as a "safe and suitable choice" that should be "available to more women."[2]

In essence, it was a hospital birth…and dumb luck…that lead me home.

# All Packed

Wade, bless his heart and per my ob-gyn's instruction, packed my "tunneling wound" twice a day for weeks.

He is a big dude. Not to sound too stereotypical, but like many big dudes his tolerance for bodily fluids is anything but big. The first meconium poop-filled diaper he changed was seemingly prankish and comical. It went something like this: Open diaper. Groan. Close diaper. Huuurgehhh! Open diaper. Growl. Close diaper. Huuurgehhh!

"Do you want me to get it, babe?" I chuckled lightly.

"Nope," he choked out, holding his breath. "I'm gonna do this. Just gimme a minute."

It took only one to groan, growl, and dry-heave through to the finish. Now he could change a meconium poop-filled nappy whilst eating a hamburger!

Blood, his wife's blood, and drawn open flesh proved a bit more challenging. But he did that, too.

The knot that formed above and pulled askew and forced a half-inch opening of the right side of my incision resulted in a relatively small flat tunneling wound, meaning the flesh was open just under the skin where the knot initially formed. My tunneling wound luckily had only one "channel" that extended through my subcutaneous tissue and shaped to the size of a 50-cent piece. That 50-cent piece represented the area we had to "pack" with packing materials—strips of sterile gauze—in order to absorb drainage from the wound, which is necessary in aiding tissues while healing from the inside out.

So there we were...huffing and puffing, sweating and grimacing, cursing and arguing our way through the pain...mine physical, his psychological.

White-knuckling a sterile long Q-tip, or cotton-tipped applicator if you want to get technical, Wade's grimacing eyes focused on the fore end of the sterile gauze strip. He would start with this end, using the sterile

Q-tip as opposed to his just-washed hands in striving for "clean technique," guiding a foot of sterile gauze strip through a half-inch slit in my cesarean incision. In and out, centimeter by centimeter, he would have to "pack" the strip pushed by the head of the Q-tip into every corner of the pocket-sized tunneling wound. Imagine packing for an international flight using one carry-on as your entire luggage, and the zipper through which you must pack belongings opens only to one-quarter its capacity!

"Holy mother of Jesus, that hurts like a ..." Nope, I couldn't say it. Mom was staying with us for a few weeks while we adjusted to our new-found parenthood. Needless to say her presence, especially in the wake of c-section gone bad to worse, eclipsed the need of my gutter tongue's liberation.

"I know, ba-a-abe...shit." The back of Wade's hand met his brow, wiping from it beads of concentration and worry.

"Son of a...argh." Then I was the one white-knuckling...the bed-sheet as I lied splayed out on it.

"I can't do this, dammit!" He retracted the Q-tip. "I'm hurting you."

"Don't stop! Keep going. It's gonna hurt no matter who does it. Go. Go. Now!" I coached at the top of a deep breath.

His shaky hand, that had to be willed every single time to poke sterile packing through and up into his wife's tunneling flesh, rose to the occasion working in tandem with my laborious exhales. "This is some serious bullshit. We shouldn't even be having to do this."

"You're telling me. But we are. So, go, now...'do this.'" Deep breath.

"Shit..." He readied himself for another packing poke. We had the routine down—deep inhale, long exhale, and poke, poke, poke.

"Argh!" I was groaning in anticipation before he even poked.

"Thought you said you took your pain pills."

"I did. You lie down. Let me poke through your guts. Then we'll talk. It friggin' hurts," I wheezed, having run out of air like a deflated balloon.

"If you're gonna be shitty, I'm not gonna do this anymore." He retracted the Q-tip for the twentieth time. A small tail of packing strip hung out like a tongue from a smirk chanting "na-nana-naa-nah!"

"Well, good, because we're done. Whoo!" The tongue needs to stick out, providing a "wick" of sorts in allowing the wound to drain, as well as providing convenient removal of the strip...the next time the wound needs to be packed.

"Whoo!" Wade reciprocated my relief. "I *hate* doing that." He let loose of the long Q-tip, shaking his packing hand vigorously at the wrist joint, feeling returning to it since it is free of the death grip.

"I hate having it done. And I hate even worse that I'm such an ass when having it done. I'm so sorry that we're in this position. That you have to do this. But you do it so well. You really do." I sat up, my arms embracing him, my lips nuzzling an apology on his neck.

"Don't be sorry. I'd be an ass, too. It has to hurt." His hands combed through my hair like curtain tiebacks, his lips planting tenderly on my forehead a mutual concession.

"I just don't understand any of this. Why are *we* having to fix this, babe? If someone hired me to re-roof a house and the new roof leaked, I...me...moi...would be responsible for fixing the roof, not the home-owner." My husband, born the son of a builder and a construction supervisor himself, likened my leaky post-cesarean incision to a leaky roof. He followed up with a facetious, "Do you think we'll get a refund?"

At the root of such practicality, the greater point may be this: there was nothing wrong with the roof until someone started messing with it.

Get your hospital bag packed. Then check in to L&D, where we will pack you in with a unit full of other laboring women. Birthing among other birthing women actually sounded appealing until one realizes how disproportionate the ratio is of caregiver to birthing women. We're ready! We are all packed with practices, protocols, and standing orders. None of which must first enforce common sense, unfortunately. We must immediately pack your cervix with Cervidil and later pack your veins with Pitocin. The clock is all packed, too, as progress will be mea-sured by it. We're ready! Come on, baby, why aren't you all packed?

Ergo, when my postpartum phase involved more packing, it should not have surprised me one iota.

# More Is Less

As children, my sisters and I grew up on the East Coast. Winters were great fun thanks to the snow, but they could be brutal no thanks to the yearly bout of flu. Now, I am not comparing the flu to labor and birth… well, I kind of am.

How many of you when sick as a child willingly went to the hospital? Or did you cling to the "sick couch"—maybe situated in a far-off corner or in a spare room to keep you quarantined from the herd—with a familiar and favorite blanket, staunchly siding with Dorothy who said, "There's no place like home."

How many of your mothers had formal medical training? Or did they possess common sense, resourcefulness passed down to them from their mothers, and from their mothers, and so on.

Maybe aside from coercing a sip of ginger ale and a bite of a saltine every now and then to keep you hydrated and to help you "keep something down," your mom did not "treat" or intervene in your laboring through your flu. Maybe your mom kept track of your temperature, assessed your pain and your breathing and your pulse and your level of consciousness. So long as there were no red flags, no need for professional medical attention, your mother allowed your immune system to sprout. She let your body do what it does naturally. And she let your body do this in its own comfortable environment.

Maybe your mom rubbed your back, held you or held a cold cloth to the back of your neck or held your hair back while you retched. Your mother attended you, tended to and treated you…not the flu. The flu had to run its course. It was up to your body to heal itself of the flu. But maybe your mother's attending—being there for you—afforded the inner strength, the spiritual strength to push through the discomfort. And maybe the reward of a stronger immune system, in this case, was worth the effort…the work…the labor.

With a little formal training bolstering such common sense, how many of our mothers could have been midwives. For women, wives, mothers—midwives—provided the majority of medical care in their homes, including home births, for centuries.

Was it Mark Twain who said "common sense ain't so common"?

More appropriately, in this context I should use another quote by the late writer and humorist, "I have never let my schooling interfere with my education."

I let my schooling interfere with my education.

Contemporary medical schooling has evolved; however, it is still very much rooted in the patriarchal model. This patriarchal model has more recently aligned with and has been replaced by the "technocratic model," where man might not know best but technology does. *Birth as an American Rite of Passage* by medical and cultural anthropologist Robbie Davis-Floyd is an eye-popping, thought-provoking, in-depth read on the subject that explores this question: "Why do so many American women allow themselves to become enmeshed in the standardized routines of technocratic childbirth—routines that can be insensitive, unnecessary, and even unhealthy?"[1]

If such routines represent a medical student's primary exposure to labor and birth, it may become very natural to them that birth is something that needs to be treated, that birth is a medical process rather than a basic physiological process, that birth is a technical process rather than a process that is as emotional as it is physical.

I personally witnessed this in my BSN clinical education, where the medical and technical aspects of birth were emphasized over the physiological and emotional. Advisors made certain I saw at least one cesarean birth, advising I choose certain shifts on certain days or nights of the week that were noted for higher cesarean percentages. Yet I cannot recall any advisor ever giving me pointers on what shift I would be most likely to witness a natural birth.

And, of course, the school of hard knocks does not go unlearned by anyone. Seventy-eight percent of ob-gyns admit the threat of malpractice either "occasionally," "almost all the time," or "always, with every patient" influences their thinking or action in treatment of patients.[2]

This influence only provokes "defensive medicine" wherein treatment is not necessarily the best option for the patient but "an option that mainly serves the function to protect the physician against the patient as potential plaintiff."

Many obstetricians, who pay some of the highest malpractice insurance premiums due to their "high-risk" specialty, would agree that our national thirty-plus percent cesarean rate is higher than medically necessary and otherwise avoidable. However, when formal schooling, and the school of hard knocks, and a healthcare system that rewards doctors and hospitals for doing *more*, promotes such a rate in a birth culture where many view cesarean—major surgery that carries risks for both mother and child—as not only convenient but "generally safe," where exactly is the incentive to decrease that rate?

Despite the fact that pain is uniquely purposeful in birth, schooling said my birth pain was better off managed with medication. No one has to wonder why epidurals are popular. Paramount in any medical training, "pain management" is often a much appreciated, possibly dire treatment. Fundamentally, and maybe even as a matter of pride, doctors and nurses—taught if they are doing their job well then no patient's pain will go untreated—do not want you to hurt.

Even my mother, who was present at our first birth, was relieved when I threw in the towel, um, yeah, epidural, please! She birthed me and my sisters unmedicated and in a hospital, no less. She pushed through the pain, mustering her own pain management. But she did not want me "to have to go through that."

And when, three years later, I did "go through that" at home with a midwife, my mother—who was convinced I was crazy to do so and who was convinced she would have wanted an epidural in birth had one been offered—said "I never saw anything like that. That was just amazing. How she took care of you. How she brought everything right to your home. If I could go back and do it all over again, I would call a midwife, too."

Basically, I let my schooling interfere with my instinct. My instinct that values a "less is more" approach in pretty much any aspect where it may be applied.

The adolescent me, more instinctual than the grown-up me and clinging to my mother's "sick couch," trusted that a present and attending mother's support—not only specific to illness but to rearing in general—can carry a child through and over hurdles they may not have otherwise been able to conquer alone.

The grown-up me initially and instinctively thought, but would have to later learn to trust, that an attending midwife's support can carry a birthing woman through and over hurdles she may not have otherwise been able to conquer alone.

Midwives foster a "less is more" approach, viewing active management and intervention of low-risk birth as true last resorts. Ironically, this minimalist approach requires midwives to spend *more* time attending laboring women than "attending obstetricians" do, where "studies have shown that even passive, nonmedical support during labor leads to better birth outcomes."[3] Less interventions, less cesareans, less episiotomies, even less costs for low-risk women, all while simultaneously providing higher quality of care, midwives—by virtue of mindset, common sense, and evidence-based training—are more successful in helping women birth naturally because they are invested in and tolerant of women birthing naturally.

Without unequivocal evidence to support that hospital birth is safer than home birth, the only indisputable thing hospitals provide to low-risk pregnant and birthing women is more. More personnel. More technology. More medication. More intervention. More ways in which to birth. More complications.

Less is more. More is less. Which is it?

Induction, epidural, cesarean, post-cesarean hematoma, dehisced incision, tunneling wound—what more could I have had?

Furthermore, hadn't I learned to never ask a question...unless I want it answered?

# Hobson's Choice

CERTAINLY THERE ARE OBSTETRICIANS WITH AN AFFINITY FOR AND THE SKILL set to attend naturally birthing women.

In fact, there was one such ob-gyn in the hospital in which I worked.

I had to believe my position there would give me an edge in choosing an ob-gyn, as I had seen the results of their work in taking care of patients in Postpartum. To my disappointment, the one ob-gyn who I thought would be an ideal fit for me, and who I had heard through the grapevine of patients and L&D nurses was highly respected and experienced in and encouraging of natural childbirth, was not accepting new patients.

Understandably so, she had progressively been cutting back to part-time hours in preparation for her transition into retirement. For years she kept the demanding hours—an average of 60 hours a week for most doctors, I am told—required of her in maintaining a full-time practice, providing care in her office and in the hospital. For the past few years with an emphasis on work-life balance, she geared her practice away from the obstetrical and toward the gynecological where "office hours" are easier to keep.

This essential aspiration for work-life balance in the middle of a female-dominated specialty, where female ob-gyns are essential child bearers and child rearers alike, is but one of many factors of the ob-gyn shortage. A shortage that results in less than favorable caregiver to pregnant and birthing women ratios.

Without this particular ob-gyn to choose from, my choice of a natural birth friendly obstetrician seemed on the far side of shortage. It seemed nonexistent.

Ever heard the phrase "Hobson's choice"? I had not until one of the ladies in our neighborhood, who Mila and I visit often on our adventure walks, used it. With an Irish accent that I could listen to for days, she used a lot of phrases I am unaccustomed to. I always enjoy the conversation and the education.

Thomas Hobson was a livery stable owner in England who offered customers the choice of either "taking the horse in his stall nearest the door or taking none at all." Thus, Hobson's choice is no choice at all.

My primary insurance, offered through my employ at the hospital, would not cover home birth or birthing center birth. It would cover hospital birth in hospitals exclusively within its "healthcare family." My secondary insurance—an alternative to the "faith-based nonprofit" hospital's primary insurance, which was designed to "improve access and affordability"—would cover birthing center birth and hospital birth outside the primary healthcare family with an additional and exorbitant deductible. "Affordability"?

Furthermore, the hospital in which I worked did not offer in-hospital midwifery services at the time. The only midwifery care supported was patient transfer from the local birthing center to the hospital, ultimately transferring care to an obstetrician. A competing hospital system in the area did offer midwifery services and had granted hospital privileges to midwives for the past five years. Again, my primary insurance would not cover a birth at those competing facilities.

Just spring for a home birth or a birthing center birth, my subconscious or intuition or both suggested, as evidenced by my Googling both types of providers in the area. To which my logical or fiscal sense or both asked what's the sense of having and contributing to insurance if you're not going to use it?

I must acknowledge that my primary insurance was reasonable at that time. Reasonable premium, deductible and split/cost-sharing. Basically it was before the Affordable Care Act went into effect. Ironically enough, had we birthed after the ACA went into effect, the unaffordability to me and my family could have easily secured an out-of-pocket home birth, which then would have been the most affordable option to us by thousands. And, of course, in hindsight I should have gone with my instinct and paid out of pocket for a home birth altogether. Taking into account our portion of the hospital cesarean and the additional time, money, and grief in healing from the complications of that cesarean, an out-of-pocket home birth would have been the most reasonable choice by far.

I did, however, choose to look for the bright side.

Maybe there are L&D rooms in the hospital with birthing tubs! There were not. Maybe they will let me bring in a rented birthing tub! They would not. I really wanted the tub. Water, a cool pool or a warm tub, was particularly attractive throughout my pregnancy and a necessity in the latter weeks. Its heavenly weightlessness offered comfort and rejuvenation to my pregnant bones and muscles. I could only imagine how it would aid in pain relief during labor. And I would go right on imagining, as not even that was a choice.

I did consider a doula. Maybe the hospital would provide such support. They did not. Maybe my ob-gyn's group had doulas on staff. They did not. Maybe my insurance would cover a doula's services. They would not. I could have hired an independent doula. The hospital would allow that. I was free to bring with me anyone I wanted to my birth. Then I would be back to paying out of pocket for a doula. If I am going to do that, I may as well just go the midwife route, for it would be the same cost comparatively.

Impatient with indecision and tired of making choices that were not fully supported, I finally settled on Hobson's choice. In your life you *have* done more with less choices, I heartened myself.

In accepting and taking what was available to me in the form of my primary insurance and my second choice of ob-gyn, I proceeded, feeling about those "choices" the way I felt about how I would give birth in general—wishy-washy.

Don't get me wrong, the ob-gyn I ended up with is a kind and decent, knowledgeable and likable person. She is a member of a well-established and very busy ob-gyn group. Certainly there are women pleased with the care she provides. And she was upfront with me about her birth ideology. Although I failed miserably at discerning it then.

Robbie Davis-Floyd said, "I have long believed and have stated many times in my oral presentations that the most important determinants of the outcome of a woman's birth are the attitudes and ideology of her primary caregiver(s)."

When I told my ob-gyn "I'd like to try and birth naturally," her response was "Yeah. Sure. We can give it a try. Just know, there's no need to be a hero."

Have we worked so hard at tolerance and support of choice for epidural that we have left no room for equally nonjudgmental acceptance of choice that does not involve one?

There is a question that truly fascinates me—Is it more feministic to labor with pain or with pain relief? First-wave feminist activists in the 19th and early 20th centuries demanded access to pain relief in childbirth as a woman's right. Second-wave feminist activists in the early 1960s-1980s opposed, calling for a return to female-controlled, non-medicalized natural childbirth. Third-wave feminist activists in the early 1990s-2010s opposed that opposition, revalidating a woman's right to a technological, pain-free birth, even questioning what is "natural." Isn't vaginal birth, even if under epidural anesthesia, natural? Are we presently experiencing the fourth-wave?

One thing is certain: the debate labors on. Is one more liberating and/or empowering than the other? The only unambiguous answer is that to have the choice *is* liberating *and* empowering.

If only it were that cut and dry.

"There's no need to be a hero." Heeerooo...heeerooo...heeerooo... the word echoed in my midbrain long after I left my ob-gyn's office. Was I trying to be a hero? Because I wanted to try and birth naturally?

Does it feel right? Intuition is a powerful and necessary guide.

And I ignored intuition? Something as somatic, of my flesh and in my flesh, as birth? It's like my body and my bones knew better than my birth attitude and ideology. They knew better what type of caregiver would best align with me. Why else were "naturally" and "home" and "midwife" my knee-jerk reactions when I found out we were pregnant? At thirty-six weeks I was still Googling FAQs on the local birthing center's website, wondering if I should call them to find out if they would consider me for a "late transfer."

Instinct had to grow tired of my incessant pleading over the course of a year after our hospital birth. There were not enough "I'm sorrys." You couldn't have given me enough "I wish I would haves." What I really wished was that instinct could help me understand why I ignored her and instead banked on the hospital/medical system. Even more disadvantageous, I banked on everything working itself out without putting in the work. I was not prepared. I did not understand the value of preparation in natural labor and birth.

Neither did my ob-gyn, as she tried to tell me. In not so many words, she even showed me. Her one-page "patient information list" included neither reading on the subject nor integrative natural childbirth preparation methods nor classes, but was a rundown of ultrasound, lab, and fees and payment schedules.

Interestingly enough, had I followed instinct to the midwife who attended our second birth, I would have been prepared because "preparation" is her first requirement for any birthing woman. Her 15-page "client information packet" included not only a schedule of free childbirth classes but a "client reading list" where, along with many others, books one and two were *Ina May's Guide to Childbirth* and *Birthing From Within*.

In my humble opinion, reading these revealing and revolutionary books would bode well for any woman who thinks she may want to birth naturally, and for any woman who is convinced she does not. Hobson's choice, anyone?

# Not Even A Fingertip

I LOST MY MUCUS PLUG AT TWO-THIRTY IN THE MORNING.

Unsure of whether I would be able to identify a "mucus plug"—having heard some are noticeable, some are not—I was surprised when losing mine was so obvious.

In the latter weeks of my last trimester, the loo and I had a regular rendezvous. Two-thirty on the dot. Although this time was different. It was slick when I wiped. I flicked on the light and bugged my eyes out at the egg white-looking discharge tinged with blood. That's what a mucus plug looks like, I thought, before re-snuggling the bump against Wade's back in bed.

After waking, I phoned my ob-gyn's office and was immediately put on alert as the receptionist requested I "come in to be checked."

"Um...I was just calling to give y'all a heads-up." My ob-gyn stressed doing so at each of the now weekly checkups for the past four weeks. "I'm fine. Nothing's going on. Some light lower back aches. Nothing active."

"But you have to come in. She's gonna want you to come in."

"I was just there...yesterday, for my thirty-nine-week checkup."

"But she's gonna want to check you for dilation."

"She did that yesterday."

"Can you come in now?"

"Um...yeah, I guess. If you think it's necessary?"

"Yep, it is. See you soon!"

I showed up at the office with a twinge of excitement whirling within at the premise that something was starting and that we could meet our daughter any time now, but left with the wind taken from my sails.

For starters, my ob-gyn who I was advised would "want me to come in" and "want to check me for dilation" was not even there because she had been called out to surgery on a cesarean. The nurse practitioner, the same one who would later dismiss my navel to thighs' bruising, performed the cervical check. Not only did it hurt—it had never hurt in the past four weeks that my ob-gyn did them—it was deflating.

"I was just here yesterday," I prefaced, getting into stirrup position. "I wasn't dilated at all. And I can't imagine that has changed overnight." If the NP could read between the lines, I was trying to tell her not to get her hopes up. I had read between my ob-gyn's lines, and she was not exactly thrilled about my still-closed cervix. The last thing I needed was more disappointment, my ob-gyn's reaction already leaving me to wonder if I or my cervix was somehow inept at this birth thing.

"Let's have a look," the NP encouraged, though her finesse was nowhere near her tone.

I grimaced and retracted toward the head of the examination table. "Okay, yeah, so that hurts. It never hurt before."

"All done," she encouraged again. Her tone dropping in measure to her finesse, she continued, "Nope, not even a fingertip. Call us if anything changes."

Seriously! Shoulder nag who yells everything yelled at me to yell at her. No shit, Sherlock! I could have told you that! Tell her! You could have told her that! You tried to tell her that! She made us come in for that!

My mother and my older sister birthed in the same rural hospital just twenty-eight years apart, the standard of care en vogue at their births as varying as bell bottoms and skinny jeans. Both of their waters broke before labor. My mother's birth was not induced. My sister's was, swiftly. My mother was not offered an epidural. My sister was, swiftly. After a natural and slow twenty-four-hour labor, my mother's birth was intervened with a forceps delivery. She recalls a "skid mark" tear that was sutured. After a persuaded and hurried eight-hour labor, my sister's birth was further intervened with an episiotomy and vacuum extraction. Their births provide an example of how fascinating and baffling change in years, change in providers, change in standard of care can and does alter generations of women's birth experiences.

"I don't get it, Ma. Am I supposed to be dilated?" I vented to her as we walked into The Egg & I for breakfast. "Were you dilated before you went into labor?"

She chuckled. "I don't know. I can't recall them even checking for that back then. My water broke, we went to the hospital, they had me walk the halls...your grandmother and I walked and walked and walked...until labor got underway."

"They didn't make a big deal about your water breaking first? Before dilation? Before active labor?" The nurse in me conceding that was never a good thing. "They weren't concerned with infection? Did they want to induce?"

"I don't know if that was even something they did then. It wasn't a big deal. And my water broke first with all three of you. But, obviously, things were different then," she excused.

"Well, at least my water hasn't..." You've got to be kidding! the ol' nag yelled, as I dribbled in my leggings, standing in line for a table.

Mom had a panty liner in her purse. Although she had conquered menopause for nearly as long as she had been an empty nester, everything but the kitchen sink still resides in her "pocketbook." So on we went about breakfast and errand running, no more dribbles.

I didn't feel panicked. I didn't feel a need for medical attention/intervention. The intermittent aches, wrapping like a belt around my lower back, were becoming a bit more pronounced but still an hour apart. It was encouraging. Okay, yeah, something *is* starting here, we're gonna dilate!

Upon returning home, I called in to work as I was scheduled for a shift that night.

"Hi, Jane," I said to the charge nurse on the other end of the line.

"Brooklyn?" she replied, the upward inflection already questioning my calling in. With only two more shifts on the books until my official maternity leave, we were all wondering if I would make it to the end.

"Yeah, I won't be in tonight." I giggled, giddy with the thought of an impending labor and ultimately meeting baby girl.

"So, what you're saying is, we'll see you, just not in your scrubs!" The charge nurse showed off her wit, returning my excited laugh.

"Maybe! I'm not sure it'll happen tonight, but I'm calling in just in case."

"Whatcha got going on, mama?" She asked, genuinely interested.

"Lost my mucus plug this morning. Noticing some light lower back stuff. Nothing active, but I think something's brewing. And I think maybe my water just broke? Well..." I started to correct myself—well, more like trickled—when she cut me off.

"Did you call your OB?" Her concern replaced casual interest.

"No, but I was just there this morning. I called about the mucus plug. They checked. I'm not dilated. I'll call them in a bit." Again, I did not feel as though a trickle was cause for emergency.

"You know you have twelve hours, right? From the time it breaks before you should be in active labor. You know this. I don't have to tell you this. You know the risk of infection goes up, right? Call your OB."

Heavy sigh. "I know. I will."

"You're admitting a section in room 263," I heard her muffled voice directing business as usual in Postpartum. "I gotta go, hon. Twelve hours. Call. Your. OB."

I did, unfortunately. She was out of surgery and persuaded me back to the office I just left three hours ago. The litmus paper tested positive for amniotic fluid.

I knew what was coming, having read it one too many times in patient charts.

She was not swayed by my differentiating between a gush and a dribble. Amniotic fluid is amniotic fluid. Lower back twinges, which I took to be early signs of labor, did not help my case either. And yet again, my cervix was the whipping boy. It was high, it was not soft, not effacing, not dilating…not even a fingertip!

She prescribed that we give it a "push." Of course. The plan was to beckon Wade from work, meet up at home and pack our hospital bag, then report immediately to the hospital where we would be admitted to L&D for induction.

Talk about a day of ups and downs, emotional flip-flopping. The dawn of my first birth should have been celebratory in a cool and magical manner, not tainted with angst and rush and worry. Instinct wanted to be listened to. I wanted to support her.

I did not hurry home. I did not panic or rush Wade when I called him. I talked calmly, "That's what they want to do. I don't know. There's no need to drop everything, babe. Finish up what you're doing. We'll get it figured out when you get home." In the privacy of my truck, I could hear instinct.

A few hours later and in the solitude of my shower, I could hear her more. The hot water never felt so good on my lower back. I wanted a bath. I wanted to submerge my entire full-term body into it. I did not, because my ob-gyn warned against it. A bath in the event of my water breaking would further increase an already increased risk of infection, she said.

I wanted that birthing tub, the birthing tub the hospital did not have and would not let me rent/bring in. I never felt so good being home, chances of natural labor and birth greater the longer I stayed home. Any—although not many—of the naturally birthing women I spoke with, as their nurse in Postpartum, advised "Stay home as long as you possibly can" when asked if they had any pointers on achieving a natural hospital birth.

I knew of a lady who used to be a doula. I had been going to her for eyelash extensions up until I was too far along to lie comfortably on my back while having them done. Maybe I should call her, I distinctly remember thinking whilst hemming and hawing and stalling and meandering about the house. She is open and awesome and resourceful, a straight shooter.

What would a doula do? Would she have me listen to instinct

and stay home as long as possible? Or would she have me listen to my ob-gyn and go along with the induction? Providing continuous labor support either way?

Too bad I wasn't aware of the evidence that indicates doulas are effective advocates for and supporters of naturally birthing women in hospitals. That a woman in birth with a doula has a decreased incidence of medication and intervention and cesarean, and an increased satisfaction with the birth experience overall. Or else I might have called her instead of passing it up with the thinking that it's a fine time to consider seeking a doula's help now!

My ambivalence and unpacked hospital bag must have led my mother and my husband to wonder if I had lost the gravity of the moment.

"Shouldn't we be going?" They asked, almost in unison.

"We're staying home." Oh, you wanna listen to me now! Shoulder nag who yells everything mirrored my own thinking as instinct finally spoke her truth to Mom and Wade.

To which they both said, "Home!" As in, *Are you crazy!*

I laughed. I wasn't crazy. I had simply and finally made up my mind. And it felt good. I felt good. I was going to dilate. "Yes, home. For the night. We'll get some rest and see what happens."

"But I thought you said she said we should go now, get *it* going?"

"We will go…when we need to."

My ob-gyn was obstinate about *it*.

At the end of the business day, her office called to inquire why we were not checked in at the hospital. I guess I didn't consider that they could and would follow up on such things. When I explained to the RN on the other end of the line the same thing I explained to Wade and Mom—that it makes more sense to stay home, sleep…get some rest, rather than be up all night laboring, *right*—the RN told me she would call me *right* back.

Although it was not the RN who called back.

# Insufficient Knowledge

THERE WE WERE CHECKING INTO THE HOSPITAL AND UNDERGOING INDUCTION at evening shift change, of all possible times—the worst kind of patient.

You yellow-bellied buffoon! the ol' nag yelled just before the door to our L&D room closed. She knew she was locked out. This was not the room for inner voices. This was not the room for critical nags whose outbursts could prove maladaptive to the premeditating and medicating environment.

The admitting nurse attempted to accommodate my wishes for a natural labor. She made available to me a birthing ball, a heating pad, and she pointed out the shower should I desire it, considering a birthing tub was not an option. My thankfulness for such resources overshadowed how terribly scant they were. Resources be damned, I was going to do this—sail through labor. The ol' nag should have added "half-witted" to her list of insults.

In checking off standing orders, the admitting nurse attempted to make them convenient. The fetal monitor was portable though still cumbersome, and the IV was saline-locked—inserted and capped-off for later use—so I could maintain mobility, conducive to active natural labor.

What natural labor? Everything being done centered around the primary and literal "order" of business to insert a synthetic—by definition "unnatural"—cervical ripening hormone, otherwise known as Cervidil, up into my vagina until it coated my cervix, where it was supposed to "help dilate the opening of the uterus."

I say "supposed to" because it didn't. Not even after twelve hours of labor. Still zero, zip, none, nada centimeters dilated. Not even a fingertip!

What the Cervidil did do was interrupt a progressive and natural pattern of early labor that was gentle and manageable, a pattern I could have slept through with the occasional waking until active labor began.

Instead, due to Cervidil, we were up all night attempting to manage an increasingly unmanageable induced labor pattern.

I would not know until my home birth how very different naturally occurring contractions feel from artificially persuaded contractions. I would not know how the first are more user friendly than the latter. I would not know how to manage contractions until I prepared to manage contractions, period.

I just kept thinking, Holy Good God, how do people do this? People do this. Women do this, all the time. I should be able to do this. Why the hell can't I do this?

Contractions getting the best of me, being up for at least twenty-four hours and laboring for the last twelve, and finding out I still hadn't dilated...my determination was caving.

Seven o'clock in the morning, it was time for IV Pitocin. That is the protocol—twelve hours. So strange, everything in the hospital is timed. I knew it then, as a nurse, but never gave it any thought. Who would have known that three years later, and in the afterglow of a natural home birth, a clock on labor would seem as absurd as a clock on menses, urination, defecation, orgasm, all things for which the anatomical, physiological, hormonal feedback loops are necessary and responsible in achieving. Sure, busy couples may have to schedule lovemaking, but does anyone actually time it!

But right there in front of my hospital bed, in front of my face, in front of my consciousness, on the unfeeling concrete wall was a large clock. Not a digital clock. A traditional black on white, stark contrast, attention-grabbing clock with a ticking second hand by which everything was measured: if Cervidil insert is ineffective after twelve hours, then proceed with IV Pitocin.

Doesn't it just make you want to ask why twelve hours? Is that the magic number?

So many questions I would ask now, in hindsight. Why are you so concerned with risk of infection due to ruptured membranes yet you don't think twice about prescribing to me, a woman in her mid-thirties, Cervidil that, according to the manufacturer, should be "exercised with caution in patients with ruptured membranes" and "use in women aged thirty years or older may further increase the risk associated with labor induction"?[1]

Who decides which is the greater risk? Infection or induction?

I believe Robert Frost made mention of it first, but I like Jay Parini's example: "We proceed on insufficient knowledge, trusting in what comes, in what comes down in winding corridors, in clamorous big rooms, above a gorge on windy cliffs."

With an overabundance of knowledge/standing orders/standard of care, we proceeded on insufficient knowledge and trusted in that "clamorous," if anything, "big" hospital room...and it failed me.

Not long after starting IV Pitocin, which made contractions even stronger—slamming would be a more appropriate characterization—than Cervidil, my resolve for an unmedicated birth was no more.

Hunched over into position on the side of the bed, I gritted my teeth through contractions growing insufferable while having to sit as still as I could as an anesthesiologist threaded a catheter into the epidural space of my spinal cord.

Though risk was regulating my birth, how strange no one would question...risk associated with epidural. It wouldn't be recommended or provided if not generally safe, if benefit didn't outweigh risk, right?

Curiously, the many risks and side effects to both mother and baby associated with epidurals are not as widely shared, elaborated on, made known as the benefits. One of the greatest benefits, indeed, is to the staff. Pain management complete, check! And, frankly, it frees up time. Critical to an already outnumbered and oft overworked personnel, a laboring woman in pain may require more tending to, more guidance, more one-on-one attention.

Or is it overexposure that numbs ears from taking seriously the laundry list of risks? Imagine the customary and ever-airing drug commercial, complete with off-screen and run-on voice, where the rundown of side effects takes up the majority of costly ad time. Does anyone actually catch all, let alone take heed, of such lists?

Or perhaps it was my egotism that underestimated the side effects ever pertaining to me.

Studies show that epidurals can cause and/or persist an already occiput posterior—"sunny-side up"—positioned baby.[2] OP labor, where
baby is face up instead of face down, meaning the hardest part of
baby's head rests on mom's lower back instead of belly, is often notori-
ously long and accompanied with back labor. Back labor akin to Public
Speaking 101, nobody wants to sign up for it.

I had no idea of the association between epidurals and persistent
OP position. I had no idea that baby girl was in OP position…until it became the general consensus between assigned nurses that OP position
was the probable cause of my back labor.

My ob-gyn had never mentioned OP position, or any other position for that matter, at my prenatal appointments. She never palpated
my abdomen to find out either. "That's what we have ultrasound for!"
she said cheerily at one appointment when I asked if she could show
me "how to tell where baby was and what part was what." I expected
if anyone could, she could. A doctor of obstetrics and gynecology, a
doctor of all things female/reproductive/fetus, if she could not palpate,
then who could?

I would later discover in a subsequent pregnancy and birth that
midwives palpate. Mine did. And it made all the difference.

Nonetheless, I felt a surge of hope when I saw my ob-gyn—the first
doctor I saw in the hospital and twenty hours into an induced labor. By
the time I saw her, I was in no position to advocate for a position. After
the epidural took effect, I slept. I don't know if it was sleep deprivation
or drugs, or a combination of the two, but I had to battle keeping my
eyes open.

She checked me for dilation. Still zero, zip, none, nada.

Further deflating but not surprising, seeing how the Pitocin drip
was pretty much useless, barely running, as baby girl was not a fan.
Every time they would try and dial it up, the fetal monitor would show
heart decelerations. Heart decelerations that would resolve once nurses
encouraged me to reposition to left-side lying position. They also had
me hooked up to oxygen on and off as a precaution to make sure baby

girl was getting enough. How could she with me lying on my back, half comatose, in bed?

What a mess…that is all I can think, looking back on it now. An unnecessary mess.

Knowing Mila, dearest daughter would have come…in her own sweet time. Independent and generally curious yet cautious of everything, Mila responds best to having a choice. Her choice. Just like her daddy, as a curious yet cautious boy, once told his Memaw when she commented on how slow he was going in his go-cart, "I do slow good."

But there we were augmenting her descent and wondering why it wouldn't add up. According to the monitor, because they always have the answers, contractions were great. They had been great—long, strong, regular—falling within "active" labor guidelines, yet I had not dilated.

My ob-gyn tried manual cervix stretching. She referred to it as popping. "I'm going to try and 'pop' your cervix," I distinctly remember her saying.

The hows and whys unaddressed, I did not request they be explained. Why start questioning now? This trust—proceeding on insufficient knowledge—happens a lot in medicine, in labor and delivery expressly. It is a vulnerable time, laboring and birthing.

Later I would learn manual cervix stretching is sometimes done in an attempt to soften and dilate the cervix. However, it is *not* ideal on a cervix that is high and closed, such as mine was. Basically, the only effective thing manual cervix stretching did in my case was provide false hope. By providing a manual number of dilation, it established a bar of expectation that ultimately led to more frustration.

"Ah, there we go!" My ob-gyn's "pop" garnered five centimeters of instant dilation. Finally!

The positivity helped shake me from lethargy. We were back on!

Just in time to find out that my ob-gyn would be off…for the rest of the night. Even though it *was* a Thursday night. Thursdays being her routine on-call assignment, as we had previously discussed in a hypothetical "what are the chances of you being at my birth" conversation.

"Just make sure and birth on a Thursday and I'll be there," she had said.

I had chuckled and replied "Oh, I'll get right on that," figuring if such were the case then Thursday would be the last day on which I would birth.

Another stroke of "dumb luck"? Here we were birthing on a Thursday and she had to excuse herself home, sick with the flu.

"What do you mean you're leaving?" Wade asked, possibly the only question he asked in our labor and birth.

"I have a fever. I don't want to be contagious to anyone," my ob-gyn explained, responsibly. "Besides, the way I feel, I wouldn't be of any help to anyone, anyhow."

I could see the bewilderment on Wade's face. You mean doctors, like the rest of us, are not immune from having lives of their own? They are not immune from commitments that take priority over the hospitals they work in and the patients they treat or work on? Doctors must first take care of themselves?

It is not wasted on me that my ob-gyn and I had our very own episode of trading places, that she was where I should have been—at home—and I was where she should have been—in the hospital—on the night of my first birth.

It would take this mix-up, the result of this mix-up, to assure I would be in the right place for my second.

# The Average Woman

I SPENT THE NEXT HOURS ON HANDS AND KNEES IN THE BED. NOT KNOWING why exactly, it hurt less when I did. Even with the epidural, I had lower back pain with contractions. Was it wearing off? Was it misplaced? Was my body building a tolerance to it? Whatever it was, it was not providing complete pain relief. My left leg was the only thing that felt numb, unable to stand on it. But I could kneel on it with the help of my arms and right leg, which weren't numb at all and had full range of motion.

Eventually I asked that the epidural be removed altogether. With the IV lines, the urinary catheter tubing, the bulky monitor strapped to my belly, being confined to the bed, my numb left leg, the fact I could still feel contractions on some level—the displeasure was snowballing. Could I just hulk out like the big green guy and rip from my body everything that was not naturally attached to it and heave the whole lot out the window?

"Oh, that would be a very bad idea," the anesthesiologist agreed with the nurse. "The line is already there if we need it later (i.e. cesarean). Your body's natural pain relief pathways have been disrupted for as long as you've had the epidural. You take that out and it's gonna be pain magnified by ten."

That made sense then, even though I did not care for the answer. It makes greater sense now, after laboring naturally at home, able to acclimate to the flow and intensity of contractions as they built. The rhythm is necessary, perfectly designed. Cutting off the epidural cold turkey after hours of relief would have been a shock to my system. Talk about hulking out!

At shift change, I saw the second ob-gyn since I had been admitted twenty-four hours earlier. He, being the on-call ob-gyn who would ultimately perform the cesarean, checked me yet again for dilation. "I'll give you a seven," he said with a smile. "Seven and a half would be generous."

"Okay, so, four hours…two centimeters," I tabulated from the previous five centimeters established via manual cervix stretching. "That's not bad, right? It's two more than before and it took forever to get there." I chuckled, feeling optimistic that at least we were progressing.

"Well…" he paused, "…the standard is one centimeter per hour."

And there came deflation once more. One centimeter per hour? Good Lord, I should be like twenty-four centimeters by now!

"But I'll give you some time. First, let's try something," he encouraged.

The something he tried was "turning" or "spinning" or "manual rotation" of baby from posterior to anterior position. He instructed me to lie in Trendelenburg position—feet elevated fifteen to thirty degrees higher than head—where I would bear down and push while he attempted to "turn" baby. This would be the only time I would push in my entire birth.

The turning didn't work. Baby girl didn't budge.

Nevertheless, shift change brought with it a particular night nurse whom I really appreciated. She stayed in the room with us, spent time with us.

"You're doing good. Stay on your hands and knees. That helps with back labor." "Flip-flop from your hands and knees to left-side lying. And when you're in left-side lying bring your right knee to your chest." "Here, I'm going to change your bed so that it's more upright. You stay on your hands and knees. We'll try and maximize those contractions. The uterus tilts forward during contractions, so a more upright position can help."

There I was, renewed with hope and feeling like an amateur rock climber on hands and knees on an inclined bed, asking in befuddlement, "How is this the first I'm hearing any of this?"

She shrugged, apologetically.

Is it because I'm a nurse? A postpartum nurse? Not a labor and delivery nurse. A part-time postpartum nurse for the better part of a year, still a bit of a greenhorn to the specialty. Do they think I know this? Because I don't.

I babbled sort of repeatedly and said, "I didn't know any of this. You're the first person to tell me any of this. Thank you. And you're here with me. Spending time with me. Thank you."

No surprise, being active and purposeful and supported, time flew. The on-call ob-gyn was back to recheck dilation when it seemed as though he just left. And he kind of did, just two hours ago. How was it I had been here twenty hours before seeing my ob-gyn, before seeing a physician, period, and here he was twice in a two-hour timeframe? Now was the time? The clock had stopped? In two hours? Two hours into labor with this invigorating night nurse?

According to my previous calculation—two centimeters in the last four hours—I was hoping for a centimeter, one measly centimeter. Come on, eight!

Well, shit. Still seven. Even after being more active, as active as I could be with the epidural in my back.

Then PROM came up again. Not the one where I unfortunately and unfashionably chose to wear a Southern belle type dress and big hair, but my "premature rupture of membranes"—PROM—where the membrane of the amniotic sac and chorion rupture more than one hour before the onset of labor. However, much like my Southern belle/ big hair prom, this PROM had a curfew, too. At thirty-six hours into PROM, I was already twelve hours over curfew, told and believing the risk of infection goes up exponentially beyond twenty-four hours.

"The biggest risk is chorio, obviously," the on-call ob-gyn said.

"Chorio" is medical jargon, an expeditious and more pronounce-able way to explain chorioamnionitis: inflammation of the fetal membranes—amnion and chorion—due to bacterial infection, typically resulting from bacteria ascending into the uterus from the vagina and is most often associated with prolonged labor.

Choooriooo…choooriooo…choooriooo…the diagnosis echoed in my head. What I knew of chorio was enough to make my blood pressure spike with the thought of baby girl in NICU instead of in my arms, with the thought of IV antibiotics running through her precious newborn veins. No, no, no. That cannot happen.

"Okay. One more hour. Can we have one more hour?" I asked, to which he agreed.

I don't know what the hell I thought was going to happen in an hour. A miracle? I don't know that I was thinking at all. Looking back, it is quite evident I was motivated by one consistent thing from the time my water trickled, my ob-gyn's response to my water trickling more precisely, through the next thirty-six hours. And that motivation was the most powerful motivation of all...fear.

I bought into it, regrettably, fear-based decisions that played right into fear-based medicine.

I was in the hospital, not the voting booth, wasn't I? Operating out of/capitalizing on fear—Does one select the treatment/candidate one thinks would be the best? Or does one select the treatment/candidate one thinks would be the least worst?

Carl Jung said, "Through knowledge, the unconsciousness is robbed of its fire." The ol' nag who yells everything, that insensitive fiery ol' bat would not have let fear rule her decisions.

How could I know so much yet know so little? PROM does not equate to chorio. Chorio can occur without PROM. I was not positive for group B strep, one of many bacterial culprits that can cause chorio. I did not have an intrapartum fever. I was not tachycardic—heart rate over 100 beats per minute. Baby girl was not tachycardic. I did not have any vaginal discharge other than the initial amniotic fluid dribble.

And how, pray tell, does such standard of care make sense? Here we had this looming fear of risk of infection due to PROM yet no one feared continuing cervical checks. When the universal advisement with a case of PROM is "nothing in the vagina." How is a gloved hand, sterile glove or not, "nothing"? A gloved hand that coincides with a timed clock that only exacerbates more fear. Fear of not doing it right, fear of not doing it in time. Come on, come on, come on, dilate!

Not to mention there are studies suggesting higher rates of PROM in antepartum women subjected to standard weekly cervical checks, usually starting at thirty-six weeks, than in those who have no weekly vaginal exams. Such studies further conclude there is "no benefit" to these exams, period.[1]

Evidence now leads me to wonder if my PROM occurred naturally or was one more, maybe the initial, casualty in the cascade of interventions. Am I to believe it was sheer coincidence that I experienced PROM just one hour after a cervical check? Just one hour after a cervical check that was my fifth total to that point but my second in a matter of twenty-four hours. Just one hour after a cervical check that was painful…when others were not.

Interchangeable with the ever-popular "failure to progress"—perhaps the most preventable reason for cesarean—"arrest of dilatation" was the diagnosis chicken-scratched into my chart.

The explanation was something like you've been at seven for the last three hours, that we know of. You could've been at seven longer than that. Seven is the start of transition labor, which is usually the shortest phase, somewhere between a half an hour and two-and-a-half hours for the average woman.

Apparently I am not the average woman, I remember thinking. If I were, I would have transitioned and been pushing by now, quite possibly even holding baby girl in my arms.

Oh…

But I am…

The average woman…

One in three of us who labor and birth in a hospital will come out with a cesarean.

# What If

Twenty minutes later, baby girl was born.

Twenty-three minutes, to be exact, from delivery room to operating room to hearing her first wildcat cry.

I labored nearly thirty hours, half of that unmedicated, the other half medicated but not completely numb. Of the last forty hours, I slept on and off for six when the epidural was first placed. My cervix, plastered with a synthetic hormone and manually stretched to force an effacement it obviously was not ready for, fought for seven centimeters. For what? Why? To have my baby pulled with hands through a man-made incision in twenty-three minutes? In one percent the time I labored?

Now I can look back and accept what I cannot change. But for a spell, the very thought permeated my psyche until it physically nauseated me. For I assumed I was to give and receive something in addition to my child in birth. I was supposed to grow from the experience—the rite of passage—wasn't I? Something was supposed to come through me along with my child, wasn't it?

My unnecessary cesarean.

Baby girl was perfect, in no danger other than a scalpel cutting through the muscled organ in which she was enveloped. As my medical record read, "A vigorous female infant was delivered from the vertex presentation without difficulty."

She had great tone, great lungs. She was alert. No trouble latching, she breastfed like a champ.

We were both fine. Vital signs stable, no fever, no infection…no reason for a cesarean.

Her little coned head took a few days to round out. There was "considerable caput and molding and the infant was in occiput posterior." She was not coming forehead first, often the greatest concern in OP positioned babes, lending itself to increased risk of tearing, vacuum/

forceps/cesarean delivery. Her chin was tucked. When I look at pictures of her oblong and vaguely alien head after birth, we didn't have much further to go. We were so close.

Always and forever leaving me to wonder how things would have progressed if I had pushed for more time? And why didn't I?

Though I knew what the on-call ob-gyn recommended, what he wanted to do, what he preferred to do, it was my decision. It was my hand that held the pen that signed the consent form for the unnecessary cesarean. It was my ego that did so without a second thought to the laundry list of complications. It was my ego that thought the "could happens" did not apply to me.

To his credit, in telling the whole truth he even said, "It's up to you." The nod of advocacy followed up with "I just want you to be aware that I have four others who are looking at sections. And I strongly feel that's where we're headed." Standing at the foot of my motorized hospital bed in signature surgical scrubs, a face mask tied about his neck, he continued "We can go now (before the storm, I supposed). Or I can come back later." And again with another, "It's up to you."

It was up to me. Not only the cesarean but the months-long fallout and healing—physical and emotional—thereafter. Clearly, closure was up to me.

I get it. She, he, no one could have said "I'm sorry." In certain states, certain laws and lawyers have been successful in using those two words against healthcare providers, doctors particularly, in establishing guilt. Yes, disturbingly, healthcare providers are sometimes punished for being candid with and empathetic toward their patients.

Even so—and with no malice, no accusation of malpractice—an "Aw, man, that really sucks. I hate that that happened" would have provided something...closure, maybe, from the one who literally opened it.

In search of that closure, I spent far too much time with questions for which there were no answers:

What if I had waited? Refused the cesarean altogether.

What if I had known thirty hours was not necessarily long, neither exceptional nor dangerous, for a first labor?

What if I had stayed home longer? Labored on my own without induction.

What if I had refused the induction altogether?

What if I wouldn't have gotten the epidural? It is proven they, accompanied with induction, can and often do cause a cascade of interventions.

What if I would have waited longer to get the epidural? At least until I knew I had dilated somewhat. Data supports that epidurals in early labor, before baby has a chance to rotate and/or "come down," persist OP position.

What if my water hadn't broke?

What if I had refused weekly cervical checks, specifically the one that hurt, the one where my water trickled a short hour later?

What if I had known the research that supports effective management of "full-term PROM" without induction? That PROM, in and of itself, is no reason to flip out and start the timer.

What if I had known one in every five OP pregnancies will have a rupture of membranes before the onset of labor?

What if my ob-gyn had performed routine abdominal palpation and educated me on exercises, both postural and positional, I could have done to try and help baby scoot to the anterior during pregnancy and labor and birth?

What if I had a different ob-gyn altogether? An ob-gyn who understood and advised me, empowered me with informed decisions rooted in evidence-based practices, such as there are few what-ifs in healthy low-risk, full-term birth; that PROM alone is not one of those what-ifs. An ob-gyn who had the aptitude to intervene when necessary, but more importantly the aptitude to know when not to.

What if my insurance would have covered birth at a different hospital? Studies show the hospital, and its policies, has a large impact on the type of birth a woman has.

What if my insurance would have covered birth with a midwife…in a hospital, in a birthing center…at home? Evidence shows women under the midwifery model of care feel informed, supported, prepared, positive overall about prenatal care and birth experiences and outcomes.

What if? What if? What if?

It could drive a woman batty.

Then I think about obstetricians, their daily practices revolving around what-if, risk, fear. What must it be like for them? What must that type of pressure do to them? To their practice? How can they—let alone their clientele—feel informed, supported, prepared, positive overall about prenatal care and birth experiences and outcomes? In a perpetual environment of what-if? *If* such is the case, I feel for them. There must be a better way.

My perpetual what-if environment relatively short-lived from the time my water dribbled to about eight months postpartum when physical and psychological wounds fully closed, I can neither imagine routinely living in, working in, making decisions in that space, nor would I wish it on anyone. Indeed the most magical moment of my life—a newborn, being a new mother—the "what-if" tainted that.

It would not dawn on me how my postpartum what-if stint was only natural. It was too miserable. I spent too much time suppressing it until I could fully escape it. To realize how the energy, the motivation, the sentiment with which we start things—my labor and birth very much starting with what-if—is often precisely how those things are carried out.

# What More

As if asking "what if" was not enough torture, I had to ask "what more."

Upon the initial and diagnostic hematoma visit, as a preventive measure my ob-gyn prescribed a hefty dosing of antibiotics. Free from fever, the blood draining from my wound free from foul smell, free from infection for the past week, I instinctively thought, why antibiotics now?

With my medical training knowing full well the answer, apparently the nurse in me conceded to the preemptive measure as I heard myself ask, "Should I take a probiotic while on the antibiotic?"

I didn't know much about probiotics other than I heard of them being recommended in conjunction with antibiotics. I didn't know much about antibiotics either. Sure, I learned of them—classing, dosing, therapeutic action, indication, side effects, et cetera—in nursing school. As an ICU nurse, I administered my fair share of antibiotics to patients pursuant to doctors' orders. I had taken the occasional antibiotic, free from any associated side effects, for the occasional persistent "bug" that seemed to need shaking.

But I was not aware of how unheathful they can be, instead assuming they were always healthful and necessary when and as prescribed. Why else would they be prescribed? "Antibiotics changed the world." "Antibiotics are the foundation on which all modern medicine rests." To quote Megan McArdle, "Life without antibiotics would be nasty, brutish and short(er)."[1] Though they do not come without consequences, I am learning, as most any synthetic thing made to imitate a natural product falls short of nature's naturally symbiotic relationship. And nature fights back, habitually winning by progressively outsmarting that which derives from imitation—à la antibiotic resistant "superbugs."

Was my ob-gyn unaware of such repercussions? Surely not.

But why then did my ob-gyn answer, "The probiotic is not necessary. There is no conclusive evidence on whether probiotics are effective at all."

And I listened to her, went against that little voice inside me—or the loudmouth who yells, rather—once again. Why did I keep doing that? If probiotics seemed to me a sound idea, somehow weaved their way into my awareness, why didn't I pursue probiotics? Seek a second opinion, ask around, ask a pharmacist, Google it for crying out loud!

The initial antibiotic prescription was for two weeks. That two weeks went by and we were still packing the wound, so she prescribed it for another two weeks. Then, a week and a half later, she said we could stop packing and stop the second prescription because the inside of the wound was healed. We just needed the exterior skin—the half inch part of the cesarean incision that popped open—to close.

"You mean I don't need to finish the prescription completely?" I asked.

We were taught in nursing school, and educated as nurses to educate our patients, that if an antibiotic regimen is started it should not be interrupted but finished "as prescribed" even if the patient is "feeling better." Otherwise improper or interrupted consumption of an antibiotic prescription before it is "gone" is possible cause for rebound infection or antibiotic resistant infection.

"Nope. You don't need to. You're in the clear," she responded, optimistically.

"So…just stop taking them?" I had to ask again about antibiotics prescribed to me for an open wound when the exterior skin of that wound had yet to close. "I already took my first dose this morning. I shouldn't finish them? That's okay?"

"Yeah, I only prescribed them prophylactically. So, no, you don't need to take them anymore."

"Okay. Cool!" I gave in to the optimism, always excited about not taking medication.

Three days later I was in her office with an incision infection. And the ol' nag who yells everything was on the hunt for James Lipton! I told you! I knew it! You should have finished the damn prescription! And you should have taken the damn probiotic! Would you just listen to me, dammit! Number Seven! Motherfucker!

Do you remember meeting "the one"? The one who was supposed to be the love of your life; the one who did not share in the reciprocal feeling? Then maybe you tried to move on, but you were still hung up on the one. And the poor soul who fell for you thereafter—who thought you were the one—had no idea they were "the rebound."

Well, that was my skin infection—a "rebound infection." The exterior skin of the half-inch part of the incision that was still open was infected. Caught early enough, it was just starting to redden. There was no pus, no heat, no fever. It would not require more oral antibiotics, but a topical antibiotic. A true rebound...it was nothing serious.

I may play with words, but make no mistake about it: rebound infections can be very serious. Rebound infections occur when a primary infection is not fully resolved or when a patient no longer responds as expected to prescribed antibiotics. Rebound infections can also occur when there is no primary infection, but as a result of preemptively prescribed antibiotics, as in my case. Regardless of how they come about exactly, rebound infections are notorious for coming after an antibiotic regimen is stopped, and even more notorious for coming after an antibiotic regimen is stopped prematurely.

A classic chicken-and-egg dilemma—Did starting the antibiotic cause the infection? Or did stopping the antibiotic cause the infection?

What I would later discover, upon explanation from a thorough family medicine doctor whose acquaintance I made while experiencing yet another cesarean rebound, is that antibiotics can destroy beneficial bacteria protective of the gut, the vagina, the mouth, everything inside our bodies.

Studies support that merely one round of antibiotics alter "flora," referred to as "ecology" or "microbiome" or "microbiota," which are ecological communities of commensal, symbiotic and pathogenic microorganisms found in all and on all multicellular organisms from plants to animals. These antibiotic-induced alterations to one's microbiome do not end when the antibiotic ends. It can take up to a year or longer to recover, if it can fully recover. Such alterations as reduced diversity and modified composition of gut microbiota can possibly and indirectly affect long-term health. Simply put, there is an impact on immunity, metabolism, even gene expression with the ingestion of antibiotics.[2]

The takeaway from such studies is not anti-antibiotic, but rather the treatment does not end with antibiotic. To take a medication/drug to treat one thing unfortunately does not suppress the fundamental side effects of the medication/drug. If an antibiotic is absolutely needed, it is not the end treatment. If the antibiotic is successful in treating the pathogen, the body as a whole—the microbiome, if you will—must be equally treated and for a length of time that seems sensible to one's re-cuperation of microbiota.

Not all "bugs" are bad. We all have good and bad bacteria linger-ing on us and in us. Not all antibiotics distinguish between good and bad, wiping out the good with the bad. If the bad replenish themselves in greater numbers before the good, then the bad takes over—classic rebound infection. Some argue this bad over good outcome can be exac-erbated by bad over good nutritional choices.

I am going to go ahead and admit the bad over good nutritional theory likely pertained to me. Maybe not from an outside glance, ge-netics and regular exercise giving the appearance all was well. The same as I was not aware of the preparation required for labor and birth, I was not aware of the preparation required—educating myself, resourc-ing reputable and natural foodstuffs that are fed a diet natural to them, spending time in the kitchen—for optimal nutrition. Feeding myself and breastfeeding another, I did my best to follow the standard Western Food Pyramid guidelines. Which is why, in hindsight, I am certain I was nutritionally deficient. Alas, a ripe host for an antibiotic-induced micro-biome alteration and subsequent antibiotic-induced intestinal infection.

Additionally, I may as well go ahead and admit that I was unaware of the unhealthful side effects of antibiotics because I did not care enough to know. One more thing that didn't apply to me!

Uh-huh...

# Just In Case

THIS IS TOO MUCH, I AM THINKING, HUNCHED OVER A "TOILET HAT"—SPECIMEN collection container for urine and stool—and scooping my own poop with the smallest collection spoon known to man as provided by the urgent care clinic.

With gloved and shaky hand, I transport what must be the foulest smelling number two known to man into five different specimen collection tubes. All of which have stringent collection and handling guidelines, consisting of one tube that must be put on ice until delivered back to the urgent care laboratory. Fill to this line. Shake this one. But do not shake that one. Keep this one upright. Put your left foot in. Put your left foot out. Do the hokey pokey…

I am all about a good science project, but a PhD in Poo I never sought to undertake.

Oh, suck it up! the ol' nag chimed. It's not like you haven't done this before! She was right. I had. More than I cared to count as an ICU nurse, faithfully. At least this time it's yours! She yelled before letting out a raucous laugh, attempting to help me keep a sense of humor about such a humbling, nearly downright demeaning experience.

It wasn't enough that for the past three days I had kept my toilet as busy as a porta-potty at a chili fest. Now I had to scoop and scoot its contents into specimen containers that were not much bigger around than my thumb. Then I had to take said specimen containers back to whence they came, handing them over to an actual human being—a laboratory technician—who would know exactly what I had to do to fill the containers. Oh, joy.

Newly back to work from maternity leave, I came off a twelve-hour night shift, saw Wade off to his work, and spent some sweet morning time with baby girl before getting her down for a nap and before retreating to my writing desk. That is when it hit me, *the urge*.

By the time I decided to go to urgent care, collected and returned said collection, seventy-two hours had passed and so had the urge. Thank you, Jesus!

By the time the results came back another seventy-two hours passed and I had been...ahem...solid for three days. The preliminary tests were negative. Maybe it was just a gastrointestinal virus, I thought. Strange virus, though. No nausea, no aches, no pains, no cramps, nothing, except the urge.

Comparable to the fact that I never considered a cesarean, I never considered having a positive stool culture for *C. diff—Clostridium difficile.* Of all the tests they were running on my stool, that was the one I was certain it was not. You ignoramus! the ol' nag yelled. Batting zero for two, aren't you, smart girl!

*C. diff*, much like birthing, was something I knew just enough about to scare the bejeezus out of myself. As an ICU nurse, I knew that if a patient contracted it, then I and everyone else—doctors, nurses, technicians, patient family members—entering their room had to be "gowned up" with disposable smocks, masks, and gloves in accordance with "contact precautions" in an attempt to prevent "contamination." I knew that it was a growing "epidemic" in hospitals, and that it most commonly affected older adults in hospitals and long-term care facilities. Although, with incidences on the rise in "generally healthy" populations, it is now a growing epidemic, period, and a devastating one at that in certain cases. I knew that it could cause symptoms ranging from diarrhea to life-threatening inflammation of the colon. I knew that it could be very resilient, even resistant in causing reinfection, and that its "spores" could hang around for days, weeks, months on surfaces.

Needless to say, for sanity's sake I was better off not knowing what I had. I had it and was over it. It had stopped. But I was *not* "gowned up" during that timeframe. Therefore, I spent the next days, weeks, months scrubbing everything I could, drying my hands out to the Sahara, worried sick that I might pass it on to baby girl or Wade. Seriously, I lost weight under the burden of worry.

How was it I escaped contracting it as an ICU nurse in the trenches, taking care of and handling stool samples from patients with *C. diff*? How was it in a chapter of life—between the ages of eighteen and twenty-one that seems like a lifetime ago—I vaccinated, castrated, culled, roped, branded, and ear-tagged cattle where livestock stool was all around an "ungowned" me, and I never acquired anything similar to *C. diff*? How was it, in that life, I was an artificial insemination technician for cattle where my gloved hand and arm were literally shoulder-deep in a cow's bum—numerous cows' bums—in order to palpate a cervix whereby my other hand would insert a rod filled with bull semen into said cow's vagina and through that cervix to be deposited into the uterine body...and I never came down with anything such as *C. diff*? How was it in an even earlier life, my childhood on a dairy farm, I once overshot my Big Wheel into the "drop"—hollowed out section of concrete purposeful in containing cow manure—where nothing on my entire body came out smelling like a rose...and, nope, no *C. diff*, nothing like it, never ever.

Yet...I take a couple rounds of prescribed antibiotics for post-cesarean complications, and...bam!

Sitting in the office of a family medicine doctor at a follow-up appointment, I could not discern which I felt more—sadness, madness, ignorance, or gullibility.

"Always, always, always take a probiotic with any antibiotic," FM doc stressed.

"But I asked my ob-gyn that exact question," I argued, wanting her to change her tune, wanting a reason to calm down, wanting a reason for the reason I went against instinct yet again. "Verbatim, I said to her, 'Should I take a probiotic while on the antibiotic?' She said it wasn't necessary, that there isn't any conclusive evidence on the effectiveness of probiotics."

"Maybe that's because she's an ob-gyn," FM doc surmised. "I see this all the time." Maybe this is her tactful way of saying patients see ob-gyns for vaginal advice, not for advice regarding the neighbor who lives just across the perineum.

"How is it happening now? I've been off the antibiotics forever." "Forever" constituting only months in this instance, maybe this shell-shocked patient's tactful way of saying why the hell is it happening at all.

"Your case is actually quite typical," she said, maybe trying to set me at ease. It did not set me at ease. "*C. diff* can overpopulate while on antibiotics, or it can take weeks, a few months even, after the course of antibiotic treatment to gain ground. And 'broad-spectrum antibiotics,' as you received and at the length in which you took them, are the worst offenders."

Then she went on to explain the difference between broad-spectrum and narrow-spectrum antibiotics. It goes something like this: Broad-spectrum antibiotics act against a wide range of disease-causing bacteria, both Gram-positive and Gram-negative bacteria. Essentially, they are not "selective" and "wipe out" good bacteria along with bad bacteria. There is growing concern with rising "bad bacteria resistance" to them because they are so "broadly" used. Whereas, narrow-spectrum antibiotics are more selective in that they are effective against specific families of bacteria, though they too can cause side effects such as diarrhea, nausea, rash, et cetera. But overall, broad-spectrum antibiotics are more likely to wipe out normal bowel flora and allow bad bacteria, such as *C. diff*, to overgrow.

Aside from "types and prolonged use of antibiotics," I would later discover that "abdominal surgery"—cesarean—is a risk factor, too.[1] Not to mention stress. A risk factor in most everything, chronic stress wreaks havoc on the "gut-brain axis," literally stressing the microbiome and causing an otherwise stable/unstressed microbiota to become erratic and unpredictable. If ever I felt stressed, and chronically so, it was in the months following my cesarean and the serial complications thereof.

For prevention my labor was induced with medication. For prevention we birthed via cesarean. For prevention I received IV antibiotics, more medication, during cesarean. For prevention I was prescribed and took oral antibiotics, more and more medication, while healing a wound caused by a cesarean caused by an induction. For prevention—all based on fear/risk—I had taken more medication and had more medical issues in the past few months than in my entire thirty-five years. And look where it got me. Obviously medication *is not* prevention.

"In the future…" FM doc paused, maybe for effect, "anytime you take an antibiotic…take a probiotic. Don't take it at the same time as the antibiotic or the antibiotic will 'wipe it out,' too. Take it three hours or so after the antibiotic. And don't stop the probiotic once the antibiotic is gone. You want to continue the probiotic for a couple weeks, even a month or more, to replenish 'good' gut flora. That can take weeks, months, after any antibiotic regimen."

"Is there evidence probiotics are effective?" I was not trying to discount her opinion, more so attempting to reason why my ob-gyn was so quick to discount them.

"Some would argue there is not enough data or studies to say conclusively," she started. "Probiotics have been around forever, but they are in their infancy as far as how they may be of specific benefit to our gut flora, immune system, and overall health. But I have seen them work," she finished, definitively.

What I would learn, and what she was getting at, is that the term "probiotic" was not recognized in Westernized vocabulary until sometime after 1980. Even then, it was not particularly popular. Even now that the term is quite fashionable, there is much to learn. And much to debate, of course. Which probiotics—specific strains, fermented foods, freeze-dried, refrigerated, a dip in the ocean, going barefoot, making mud pies—are most effective? And for what precisely? How do they measure up to antibiotics? Is there a place for them in today's modern medicine?

Those who question conclusiveness may consider mounting evidence that points to compelling efficacy of probiotics, precisely in alleviating and reducing incidence of antibiotic-associated diarrhea by "42 percent," according to researchers who analyzed 82 randomized controlled trials.[2] Yale went one step further in singling out and giving an "A" to specific probiotic strains in the prevention of antibiotic-associated diarrhea, *S. boulardii* namely for *C. difficile*-associated diarrhea.[3]

"Dirt don't hurt," said many a mother and a father. They may be onto something: soil-based organisms. Plants thrive in healthy soil with diverse microorganisms. Do we, too?

Probiotics, through cheese and fermented foods, have been around since the ancient Greeks and Romans recommended their consumption. Remember, it was Hippocrates—the "father of medicine"—sometime around 400 BC, who said, "Death sits in the bowel." Through time and even today, fermented foods such as kimchi, sauerkraut, and kefir—packed with probiotics—were and are eaten in Asian, Middle Eastern, and European cultures.[4]

I find it quite telling that FM doc is of South Asian descent, that even as a Western medicine practicing physician she would have knowledge of and faith in, as part of her treatment plan, probiotics that by definition contrast with antibiotics:

probiotic—a substance that stimulates the growth of microorganisms especially those with beneficial properties.

antibiotic—a medicine that inhibits the growth of or destroys microorganisms.

The very contrast lending itself to the yin and yang philosophy in which it is thought that opposing forces may be complementary, interconnected, and interdependent in the natural world in order to achieve balance, growth, wellness.

FM doc's time spent informing me was much more impressive than her treating me. It didn't hurt that her integrative approach spoke to my sensibility. The notion of incorporating probiotics in aiming for the big picture of long-term health, habitually proliferating the "good" rather than simply and merely obliterating the "bad" in the now of short-term health, that seemed to me a true effort for prevention. And the collective receptivity between patient and caregiver seemed a positive example of Robbie Davis-Floyd's "determinants of outcome" riding on the "attitudes and ideology of primary caregiver" in action.

Although, no matter her faith in probiotics, FM doc too had a standard of care lawfully required to fulfill. Moments after solidifying my initial knee-jerk reaction—when instinct nudged me to take probiotics along with my antibiotics—FM doc caused that knee to literally jerk. Sitting there on her exam table, one might have thought she tapped my knee with a "reflex hammer" when she handed me a small piece of paper from her prescription pad with dosing instructions for an antibiotic...another broad-spectrum antibiotic.

"Be sure and take probiotics with this and for several weeks or months thereafter," she said.

To which I replied, "You've got to be kidding me. This is a joke, right?"

"No," she said, with an upraised brow, maybe wishing it were, "that is the treatment. The antibiotic keeps *C. diff* from growing and treats diarrhea and other complications."

"A...broad-spectrum...antibiotic to treat an infection caused by a... broad-spectrum...antibiotic?" I couldn't help but accentuate the irony, or sheer lunacy, in that. "I haven't had *the urge* in five days. Everything seems good, back to normal. Why do I need an antibiotic at all?"

Ah, yes, "Just in case."

How is it "just in case"—"for prevention"—is an acceptable reason to induce labor that causes cesarean, perform cesarean that causes complications, and prescribe medication that gets rid of one thing but causes another? And how is it that *it*, preventing one thing to cause another, has become the theme of my birthing and postpartum journey?

# Slow Learner

Unfortunately, I am not alone. The emergence of *C. diff* infection—and other infections, in general—among postpartum women directly correlates to increased cesarean rate and antibiotics used during and/or in treating postsurgical complications.[1]

In wrapping my mind around this months' long cascade of interventions, all preventable if not for supposed prevention, curiosity led me to a slew of postpartum women with similar journeys. I found them on blogs, mothering forums, breastfeeding message boards, et cetera.

Their stories stirred me in sad and infuriating yet inspiring ways, the first validation of my postpartum emotions. These women got it. They made me wish, made me pray, made me laugh as some maintained great humor about such unamusing experiences. Many humbled me, their experiences a reminder that mine could have easily been worse. All of them helped me heal, story by story, week by week, month by month, shared experience by shared experience—the impetus for sharing mine.

I tried to assimilate, considering women I knew or heard of or read about who never imagined themselves having cesareans, but ultimately did and didn't let it get them down. Women who accepted it and got on with it, no examining, no rehashing, no regret. Women who went on to have successful VBACs. Women who chose repeat cesarean for subsequent births, for a multitude of personal and medical reasons.

I clung to testimonies of women I knew—friends, nurses, ob-gyns, patients—who had both vaginal and cesarean births and who preferred cesarean or at least wished they would have had cesarean. "In and out, no muss, no fuss, I was wakeboarding on Lake Travis two weeks after all three of my cesareans." "I liked that we could plan around it." "I tore really bad in my first vaginal birth, so I was thankful not to worry about tearing again." "I had long vaginal labors. They totally wrecked my bladder. It prolapsed. I had to have bladder sling surgery. I wish I

would've had cesareans." "Cesarean all the way. I had pelvic floor surgery because of my two prior vaginal deliveries."

When I confided to my ob-gyn that my at long last healed but
cockeyed cesarean scar gave me no further trouble, except to my vanity,
she said, "You can pay a plastic surgeon to fix it, or we can clean it up for
you, when you have a repeat cesarean!"

I tried to see where they were coming from, wanting desperately to
get over my birth hang-up. Was I being ridiculous? Illogically obsessive?
Women do it all the time, have cesareans. Just because I had a less than
stellar first experience does not mean I would have another. Really, sta-
tistically, what are the odds I would have complications again. Why am
I so upset about this? The way a woman births has no bearing on who
she is, the mother she is. Birthing, in any form, does not a mother make.

But...I could not let it go.

Whether unpreparedness or disappointment or disconnect between imagination and reality, the way in which my first birth played
out left me utterly confused. Confused about who I am, about birth,
about our medical system, about my role as a nurse, about a lot of
things. No amount of cajoling or validation was going to change how
fundamentally distressing I found it, the compounding complications
and lengthy full recovery merely rubbing salt in the wound.

Aha!

Therein lies the beauty, as salt can help a wound heal faster if one
can stand the pain.

Who was it that said "There is no growth without pain"? I prefer it
said as I first heard it from a yoga instructor, "The pain will leave once it
has finished teaching you."

*That's* why I could not let it go.

I wanted—needed—this lesson.

Quintessential lifelong learner, truth seeker, cause-effect believer,
I can't help but ask "Why?" I have been doing it since I can recall. Just
ask my mother. We all want to understand the things that matter to us,
don't we? Then understanding is not enough, one must apply what they
have learned, right?

Blah, blah, blah. Just roll with the flow, would you, shoulder nag who doesn't yell everything reappeared. Hmm, where have you been? I wondered. I never left, she said, you just couldn't hear me. If she had an alpha bone in her body, she would have fleshed it out with something like, you just couldn't hear me because that bitch is always yelling.

She kept on with her calm cadence, Remember your senior term paper? Do they even have term papers anymore? Bruce Lee, what an insightful soul. "Be like water," he said, "shapeless, formless." Just chill out, breathe. You don't always have to *do* something.

But I wasn't ready to hear her yet. Poor nag, she always gets the cold shoulder. "Yet" being the operative word.

Now…now was the time to do what I do best. Organize? Plan? Prepare? Who has time for all of that? Yes, I can be that dimwitted. And the ol' nag who yells everything only encourages me—Read more! Ask more! Do more! And do it quickly, we ain't got all day!

And I did.

I started with me, the body, the vessel—who I am thoroughly convinced was galled by my signing off consent to cut it open, as evidenced by its conspiring with bad bugs and rebound infections. Get it back on track. Barefoot to the earth, get it back in touch with nature. Heal it. Engage it. Rest it. Feed it well. Encourage strength and efficiency.

A quick study, but a slow (i.e. impatient) learner, I kept reading and applying principles—and continue to do so—in an attempt to figure out what works best for me and mine and our *diet*: habitual nourishment. Like inherited birth knowledge, inherited nutritional knowledge seems almost nonexistent. In such voids, confusion and controversy reign. Is the damn egg good for us or not?

Rediscovering that knowledge, untangling the web of misinformation, making nourishing choices, and then staying on the darn wagon or at least riding the sucker six out of seven days a week—particularly in an overindulgent and convenience-driven society—*is* challenging. But further akin to labor and birth I would discover that through awareness, preparation, and following instinct, I do believe I inherently know what foods my body needs, what foods nourish and nurture it.

Such awareness and thirst for understanding and overall implementation of "wellness" rather than just fitness or health wouldn't have so much as tickled my radar if not for the unnecessary cesarean and its mishaps.

So with silver-lining gratitude—primarily to a child who gifted with her existence revelations I am still trying to absorb, secondarily to a few physicians and a medical system who collided with me on destiny's passage—I assumed I was on my way.

Heck yeah! "The pain" had to be "finished teaching me." Sayonara pain!

Uh-huh...

Hopefully hurling forward, I asked and read and watched and did it all some more. Friend, stranger, birth books and birth documentaries—I wanted to hear, read, see anything and everything about natural, vaginal, VBAC, HBAC, home, unmedicated, holistic, Bradley method, yoga method, midwifery method, hypno, water, and scads of other birth terms. Surely the librarian who heads up the "hold" department at my local branch would have choked me if she could have.

Yes! I committed, in my heart, to a home birth. Before I was even pregnant a second time. In regrettable but habitual cart before horse style.

What I wouldn't realize, in my rush to *do*, was that I had to commit with more than my heart. I had to commit with my body. Which I thought I was doing smashingly in my newfound wellness regimen. What more could my body possibly need?

My body would need me to *trust*...in it to do what it does.

Oh, joy. Trust *and* surrender? Two emerging concepts in my research on natural childbirth that can be as foreign to a doer as doing may be to a thinker. Trust in what? Yeah, trust it will get done because I will do it. Surrender to what? There is no surrender. There is only aiming, doing, trudging on to get it done.

Mark Twain said, "To succeed in life, you need two things: ignorance and confidence." Now those are two concepts I, and probably many doers, have in spades.

But this trust and surrender stuff…sure, I read about it in many of those birth books. Reading as far as I got, there was no real comprehension of it, no making it mine.

A childhood spent overcoming emotions, mine never mattered as much as my father's. Without opportunity to feel validated, to matter, to be a daddy's girl, though I desperately wanted to be…I guess. Disappointment after disappointment, a hard shell formed that was resentful, if not combative, of anything "soft."

What's softer than trust and surrender?

Ergo, it would take something more harrowing than a cesarean and its complications, something more practical than reading and studying to get through my armor.

It would take losing something so precious, something worth trusting and surrendering for, something so innocent to unmask my bravado, crumbling it into a million tiny pieces smothered in tears of guilt and resignation on the bathroom floor.

It would take losing a child—a miscarriage—to teach me how to birth another.

# II

*the learning*
*was everything but*
*felt like doing nothing*

# Biological Clock

*THIS CHAPTER, BIOLOGICAL CLOCK, RELIES ON BLOG EXCERPTS I WROTE DURING AND shortly after my miscarriage. Doing so captures the authenticity of that moment in our lives. The next chapter, Tripartite, reconvenes in present writing.*

### Biological Clock Hibernating

As a half-pint and youngest of three—my mother's baby—I never had the experience of growing up with younger siblings. Basically, I never had the experience of "playing mom." As an adolescent, I did not dream of marriage, family, children. Places, experiences, finding myself—those were my fantasies. And I spent my twenties chasing those dreams...or chasing my tail.

Somewhere between Nashville and Los Angeles aspiring singer-songwriter/wanderlust days, I found myself in a challenging but more fascinating position of teaching first grade in a school for underprivileged children outside Phoenix, Arizona. The kids were extraordinary. They were eager, energetic, blunt, charismatic, naturally hilarious, and always inspiring. For a moment, I considered staying on and pursuing education. Even then, my biological clock never ticked.

I didn't realize how good I could actually be with a child, with a baby, until my niece was born. The first baby I had the privilege of being around for any length of time and the first birth I ever witnessed, I held my sister's leg as my niece crowned and delivered. And I, the consummate "baby hog," held my niece as often as I could, convinced she would be the only baby I would ever have.

### Biological Clock Found

I don't remember the exact day. I do recall it was near the end of the month of August, as I had just returned from a seasonal massage therapist position/writing retreat at the hypnotic sanctuary that is Brooks Lake Lodge in Dubois, Wyoming. Another adventure and impromptu trip, I told myself I was there to finish another novel. I did finish the script. But a part of my motivation for the thirteen-hundred-mile trip was to try and wrap my mind around a new and budding relationship. Home base in Austin, Texas, in my mid-thirties and casually dating a man for the past few months, I could feel my not-so-casual self falling completely and inexorably in love. The thought even crossed my mind that maybe I wanted to have his babies. What woman wants to have some man's babies after dating only a few months!

Upon return from Wyoming, I accompanied said man to a peewee football game he was coaching. At game's end, the kiddos circled around him for the post-game pep talk. He was on bended knee, thoughtfully eye level with them. I am watching the kids huddled around, trusting him and smiling at him. Two kids on the ends of the circle are leaning on him, with elbows propped up on his big ol' broad shoulders. I trusted him and had come to lean on him, too. But I was not smiling. How could I when my heart was sinking with the burdensome weight of the realization that his kismet entrance into my life signified the closing of a chapter of solitary dreams. Within a few months' time, his presence—unimposing but solid as an oak—shifted my dreamscape.

A man was never an aspiration, said I. But there he was in the irrefutable flesh. Yes, I think maybe I dreamed of a life with him, complete with his babies.

Really, God? Now? This is the time you choose to put this on my heart? My first published novel and first full-length album—a soundtrack to the novel *The Boots My Mother Gave Me*—had released to some success a year or so ago. All of those scattered, unfocused, harebrained dreams of my twenties were coming to fruition. I just finished my second book, and was penning away my third. I performed regularly as part of an acoustic duo in the thriving live music scene of Austin. I even landed some out-of-town gigs, book signings, and speaking engagements. Things were finally coming together. Things that were not necessarily conducive to family life. How could I possibly be considering a family...now?

## Biological Clock Tick-Tick-Tocking

Fast forward not quite two years and not quite two weeks of official "trying," on the heels of a Maui wedding/honeymoon, I plod into my ob-gyn's office. My mind functioning in some sort of haze between poor concentration and low-grade headache, persistent nausea is my new norm. Oh, food…ugh. The only reprieve is untimely bouts of fatigue. Oh, sleep…ahh. And in those other consistent moments of unsettled writhing, trying to overpower the nausea, I secretly welcome it. Hoping it means what I think it means, fingers crossed the "stick" I tinkled on a week ago was accurate.

My ob-gyn confirms it. We are seven weeks plus one day pregnant. What! Pregnant before the honeymoon? Pregnant before we started trying?

## Biological Clock Appeased

Thirty-two weeks later and in the wee hours, Wade and I sit silently gazing at each other and at the precious bundle of seraphim sweetness coddled between us. Our soul cups fill and bubble and run completely over. It doesn't get any better than this.

I often pondered what was the big deal about being a mother, a parent? In my carefree gypsy days I would think, "Why does everybody want to do that? What's the allure?" Friends with children would say, "You're never going to understand until you have one of your own. You just don't know until *you know*." They were so right. I didn't know, completely clueless. But now that I do, that we do, there is no lovelier life than the one with her in it.

## Biological Clock Out Of Time

Nine months in, after many foibles and learn-as-you-go lessons, Wade and I somehow navigated into our parental sweet spot. Primarily, baby girl was healthy and hitting her developmental stages. We had the regimen down pat, and couldn't believe our luck—first-time parents in our mid-thirties! The joy and illumination and a host of other favorable things she brought into our lives was all the incentive we needed. Yes, we must do this again.

Six months of trying and no BFP—big fat positive—and bound to be a bit discouraged conceiving so effortlessly the first time, hope prevailed: "It will happen when it is supposed to happen."

In the meantime, I chooka-choo-choo'd my "advanced maternal age" caboose to an ob-gyn as recommended when conception had not happened after six months of trying for those over thirty-five. While it is generally recommended to try for at least a year before growing concerned for those under thirty-five. Ultrasound, pelvic exam, and hormonal bloodwork complete. Wade even had a semen analysis. Everything came back WNL—within normal limits—no medical explanation as to why we were not conceiving.

It was the first time I heard the term "secondary infertility"—the inability to become pregnant or to carry a pregnancy to term following the birth of one or more children. Although she discussed it, the ob-gyn did not necessarily diagnose us with secondary infertility. She remained positive and encouraged us to do the same, even offering a referral to a reproductive endocrinologist. We did not take her up on that. But we did heed her recommendation in using OPKs—ovulation predictor kits—to hone in on our "fertile window" in my monthly cycle.

## Biological Clock Revived

After four months of OPKs, one BFP should have brought celebration, a plethora of exclamation points and "woo-hoos." But I have none to give.

When my period was three days late, I took an at-home pregnancy test and got a BFN. I waited two more days, period still absent, and we got our BFP. Although the pretty pink line was faint. I have no idea if this should have been any indication. With our first pregnancy, the line was unmistakably positive—dark and appeared almost immediately. But it was also completed later in the sixth week. Who knows?

Bless his radiant "I'm gonna be a daddy again" heart, Wade spilled the beans to everyone. I told my mother and a few work friends, due to possible schedule changes, but preparing to wait until we made it through the first trimester to fully share the news. And I told Wade, "Babe, shhh, until we know this one is going to stick."

I couldn't put my finger on it...women's intuition, maybe...but something inside of me was unsettled. I kept waiting for the nausea to hit me like it did with baby girl. I begged it to, reading somewhere that morning sickness was a good sign of a "viable" pregnancy. I had some low-grade food aversions. Nothing sounded good one moment, everything sounded good the next. But nothing like I experienced in the first trimester of our first pregnancy. The brain fog and bouts of lethargy never hit me either.

When I shared my concerns with my mother, she offered encouragement: "Every pregnancy is different. I felt terrible with you, but I had no symptoms with your sisters. And you all turned out fine. Just thank your lucky stars you don't have to contend with morning sickness this time!"

"Thanks, Ma. Just don't go telling everyone yet." I couldn't shake the feeling that something wasn't quite right.

## Biological Clock Betrayal

I spotted for about three days at seven weeks into the pregnancy. I told myself it was okay because I spotted early on—likely implantation bleeding mistaken for a regular and light period—with baby girl. When I started spotting again at nine weeks and the spotting was not at all what I would consider benign, it was then I knew something was terribly wrong.

"Is there any possibility you could be off on your last menstrual period?" the ultrasound tech asked, her voice hopeful and reaching for positivity.

"No, Ma'am," I answered, voice withdrawn, fear realizing.

No! There is no way I miscalculated anything. For the past four months I have obsessed over tracking my cycles, stalking ovulation with OPKs, becoming familiar with things—cervical mucous, cervical position, basal body temperature—I never gave a thought to before. Everything has been checked, double-checked, triple-checked and recorded with incessant care. No! I am not off on my LMP.

"You're measuring five to six weeks," the ultrasound tech replied, her voice dropping into a soft and apologetic register. There was no fetal pole. No heartbeat.

That is when the brain fog finally hit me, a complete and horrendous cloud of surreal calamity. What did she just say? Did I hear her correctly? How can this be? *I am so sorry, baby. We wanted you...with everything within us...we really did.*

In a matter of one year, we managed to achieve engagement, tying the knot, conception, and the birth of a healthy baby girl. Maybe it was predestined, all the stars aligned? Now, after nearly one year of trying and thinking that we finally lucked out again, maybe this was predestined, too. What the hell happened to our stars?

Un-fucking-believable.

Yes. I am one of those. Foul-mouthed angry grievers. Save heart, I keep the cussing to myself, away from baby girl's ears. My anger is not flagrant, imposed upon no one. It is all for me. A slow and controlled simmer that fuels my path to survival and recovery...eventually.

"Thank you for fitting me in," I said to the ultrasound tech as she led us to the receptionist's desk. "Oh, yes, monkey says 'ooh ooh ooh eeh eeh,'" I said to Mila as she initiated me to play with her playing with a stuffed Curious George she picked out of the waiting room toy box.

My mind split between trying to focus on being a mother to the exquisitely wonderful child who stood before me in the here and now and reaching to come to terms with never having the pleasure of laying eyes on the one who stopped thriving in my womb.

Don't cry.

With murky head and shaky hand, I voided three checks before making one out correctly. Seriously! You don't have a debit card machine?

I did manage, likely out of routine, to get Mila settled into her car seat. While hugging in her arms "Potter Bear," a favorite stuffed animal, and using "Bubby," a prized blanket, as a makeshift pillow, I kissed her forehead, each cheek, nose, chin and lips. A stream of "I love yous" flooded from my mournful yet grateful mouth before I settled into the driver's seat. Five minutes of wheels on blacktop and she was out like a light, per usual the best traveler.

Now you can cry. *I am so sorry, baby.*

## Biological Clock Denounced

Wade and I tended to one another. I was not the only one it was happening to, after all. Of course, we already made plans for the tiny bundle of cells we hoped would prosper into a full-fledged newborn. A newborn who would arrive not only bearing joy but suspense at *her* or *his* birth, we predetermined to look forward to the surprise this time. Eagerly hashing over names in preparation, either way we gushed over the February twenty-ninth due date, considering it a sign of good luck. Our baby would be a "Leaper" or a "Leapling"—"a magical reputation as being lucky," so say astrologers. Could we be *lucky* enough to feel that punch in the gut, memorializing our "Leaper," only once every four years?

Life should have prepared me for the plethora of emotions miscarriage brings. It did not. The most tormenting part was reckoning with failing a precious, defenseless unborn being. Why didn't my body grow it? Protect it? Was it my age? Was it something I did? Was it karma?

If struggles are the best tools by which to learn, then *what* are we supposed to take away from this?

Is it just part of the reproductive process for some? For us? A setback? One of the facts of life?

Growing up on a dairy farm, I had a bird's eye view of those facts. Reproduction 101, it did not take long to figure out the bull mounting the cow in the pasture was not merely trying to get a piggyback... when nine and a half months later, my sisters and I watched in quiet anticipation as that same cow gave birth to a calf. It was on that dairy farm I learned about the most unavoidable fact of life—death.

As Shakespeare wrote, "Death, a necessary end, will come when it will come." Yet it does not seem just when that end comes before that life truly begins.

# Tripartite

Hᴍᴍ…

I haven't felt those emotions in a while. It is hard to believe that over time I did forget how shattering our miscarriage was. How infinite it felt, then.

And don't I feel like a drama queen now, when presumably we did not have secondary infertility at all but a benign case of impatience, when miscarriage was not the end of our fertility journey, when there are people truly struggling with infertility.

But I would do it all again. For I would not have a choice. The desire to conceive, carry, deliver, hold, love, and parent a child is as universal as it is precious. It is natural, we are told, a basic biological instinct. When that instinct, that desire, for whatever reason cannot be met, it is beyond heartbreaking. It is cruel. It is okay to feel bad, to grieve, to heal. Doing those things does not make us ungrateful. It is essential in moving on.

"Grief is not a disorder, a disease or sign of weakness. It is an emotional, spiritual and physical necessity, the price you pay for love. The only cure for grief is to grieve." — Dr. Earl A. Grollman

Akin to birthing, conventional obstetric practice may have us believe miscarriage is something that needs to be managed/treated. It, too, is under a time limit or surgery ensues:

1. If it does not pass on its own relatively quickly—the standard being up to two weeks—then medication is prescribed.
2. If medication does not assist the uterus to contract and/or the cervix to open up in expediting the passing, then surgery intervenes.
3. D&C—dilation and curettage—manually opens/dilates the cervix, where the contents of the uterus are manually removed by scraping and/or suctioning.

It seems to me another standard of care contingent upon risk/fear/what if. What if infection sets in? What if there is heavy bleeding, at worst hemorrhage? Although understandable concerns, might we consider monitoring for such risks rather than hastily performing a D&C which carries many of the same risks, such as infection and hemorrhage, and carries additional risks of its own. Just one of those risks being that a history of D&C in women is "associated with an increased risk of preterm birth in subsequent pregnancy."[1]

Depending on a woman's support system, how she internalizes the experience, and scores of other variables, it may be more humane, more beneficial to overall physical and mental health for her to seek help in expediting the process. Even though evidence suggests that there is "no difference in short-term psychological outcomes between expectant (natural) and surgical management" of miscarriage.[2]

What about the woman who is unsure of what to do exactly? The woman whose inclination says this started naturally, can't it end naturally? The woman who prefers to avoid surgery or intervention if at all possible. But who may wonder if she is being carelessly impulsive by not doing everything that is possible. The same woman who is fearing and "what if'g" already. How does anyone reason that she needs more fear and what-if?

Possibly what she needs is empowering, some evidence-based information with which to make informed decisions, such as more than 80 percent of women experiencing first-trimester miscarriage "complete natural passage of tissue within 2 to 6 weeks with no higher complication rate than that from surgical intervention."[2] Perhaps what she needs above any and all of that is encouragement...support.

I would not have realized how far a little encouragement could take me, in following instinct and fleshing out my choice, without the low-key yet steadfast guidance of a midwife.

Via word of mouth, I learned about an LM, CPM—licensed midwife, certified professional midwife—from a fellow postpartum nurse who had her children at home under the care of this midwife and who could not have been more satisfied with her birth outcomes.

I cannot say, think, write Genevieve's name without smiling, without feeling gratitude and love and nostalgia. Even Mila talks about her often, "Guess who I am? I'm Miss Genevieve, Mama." Fisher-Price stethoscope draped from her ears, the listening end pressed against the "belly" of one of her stuffed animals where she is assessing baby's "heart*beep*."

Our first official prenatal appointment with Genevieve was scheduled for week ten. One week shy of that meeting, miscarriage signs presented themselves. With the exception of a free consultation, roughly one hour in making introductions, Genevieve barely knew me. We had not made any form of payment, not even a down payment, as that would be due at the ten-week appointment.

She owed me nothing.

We were no longer technically pregnant and would not be hiring her services after all. She had already swiftly and responsibly referred me to the diagnostic group she partners with when I alarmed her of my spotting, as ultrasound is not something she does in her office. She could have just as swiftly referred me elsewhere for management of my miscarriage.

Yet she gave…her time, her support.

I did not want to be a bother, but I needed Genevieve. Without her and not far enough removed from my cesarean fallout, I knew what the alternative would be—Hobson's Choice.

Carefully choosing what seemed to be the least intrusive form of communication, I must have emailed her at least once a week. And she replied…every single time. Even when I repeated myself, my questions, my concerns. I'm sure I sounded like a broken record. Repeat. Repeat. Repeat.

It was taking forever, much longer than the "standard" two weeks. I would have a few days, maybe a week, of light bleeding with an intermittent gush or two, then nothing for two or three days, which gave me hope that it was over. Only to have more light bleeding with an intermittent gush or two for another week, then nothing for two or three days. Repeat. Repeat. Repeat.

From researching, I knew the basics of "nothing in the vagina"—no sex, no tampons, no pool, no baths—while experiencing an active miscarriage. I knew to be aware of and assess for any signs/symptoms of infection, abnormal bleeding. Of course, Genevieve reiterated this information.

What she accentuated that I needed most of all was encouragement, encouragement of *my* choice.

"Your body knows how to do this." "Listen to your body." "Be kind to your body." "Be patient with yourself." "Don't overdo it." "Rest." "Recover." "Take time to heal."

*Your body knows how to do this.*

Of all the supportive advice she gave, that one line kept coming back. That one line would get me through a miscarriage. That one line...eventually...would birth our son.

It wasn't that simple, though. The what-ifs, the fear, the impatience of my hospital birth would wield themselves in my miscarriage, too.

A month in, I emailed Genevieve about Cytotec. I had heard of the oral medication, often used in conjunction with other medications, to "stimulate uterine contractions causing the womb to expel its contents" in the event of a miscarriage. Should I try it? Could she prescribe it?

No, she couldn't recommend it. She didn't go into detail, but rather encouraged me to do my homework. In hindsight, I appreciate her fairness. She didn't go on about why she wouldn't, maybe avoiding making me feel self-conscious about why I would. She let me draw that conclusion for myself.

An interesting if not perplexing supposition, when in my homework I concluded that misoprostol—active ingredient in brand name Cytotec—may very well carry a higher rate of uterine rupture in women with previous cesareans than does VBAC in and of itself. Some obstetricians will cite this risk of uterine rupture as the reason "once a cesarean, always a cesarean" still holds. Would those same obstetricians prescribe misoprostol to a miscarrying woman who had a previous cesarean?

I wouldn't know if an obstetrician would recommend it. But I almost found out. Yes, I caved, somewhere around the start of week five and made an appointment with the ob-gyn who I consulted with when conception the second time around seemed elusive.

It was becoming quite bothersome, primarily to my psyche. So I made myself a deal by making an appointment for six weeks out. If the bleeding persists, we'll have a backup plan, just in case.

Just in case! The ol' beast roared. What if! Risk! Fear! Didn't you get enough of that! Just in case! You impatient, untrusting, pea-brained, yellow-bellied, lily-livered pantywaist!

You're the one always telling me to *do* something! I yelled back this time. My mind's interplay as combustible as dry wood, I paced the living room floor and wondered if I am the only one a few tablespoons short of a block of butter, or do other people argue with themselves, too? I'm *doing* something! I'm being proactive! I shouted again at the ol' nag.

The only thing you need to *do* is breathe, shoulder nag who doesn't yell everything chimed in, right on cue.

Oh! *Now* y'all are on the same page! I huffed back, before I laced up my running shoes and slammed the door behind me. As if it were possible to leave them—the voices in my head—behind.

Should one subscribe to Freud's "structural model of the psyche" featuring the id, superego, and ego, one could safely conclude that the ol' nag who yells everything, the ol' nag who doesn't yell everything, and I make an ideal and exasperating "tripartite."

# Storm The Castle

I WAS SO IMPATIENT.

When hadn't I been?

The moment our first pregnancy was confirmed, I couldn't wait—to get to the end of the first trimester where my nausea ended, to start showing, to tell the world, to proudly parade my bump, to get to the end of the second trimester meaning we only had the third to go, to get to the end of the third trimester and lose the bump as it grew more and more uncomfortable, to meet baby girl.

I, led by an equally impatient obstetrical/hospital birth system, couldn't wait—for her to come in due course.

Once she was here, I couldn't wait—to breastfeed her and stare into her eyes until she fell into milk drunk slumber, for her to wake again so I could get to know her for the short amount of alertness she would have before feeding and sleeping again, to bathe her, to see her first smile, to hear her first laugh, for all of her firsts.

Once we got the rhythm down, I couldn't wait—to tweak the mom-work-social life balance, to get back to gigging, to get back to writing, to get back in studio, to make the gym and Town Lake regulars on my schedule again, to grab lunch with a friend, to pump surplus breast milk for such "get back to's," even if it meant existing in a perpetual state of sub-engorgement that pumping can engender.

Then I couldn't wait—to start trying for number two.

When trying didn't work fast enough for me I couldn't wait—to enlist OPKs, to track basal body temperature, cervical mucous, cervical position, ovulation ultimately.

This was nothing new for me, the pace…the fervor.

I had a voice coach in LA who had to be some sort of a clairvoyant. The first time I walked into her studio, she watched me walk from the door and across the large open acoustic room. Her eyes semi squinting, mouth relaxed as though she may be sending an exhale through it, head tilted to the side, she said nothing.

I, uncomfortable with the silence, extended my hand over the piano she sat behind to introduce myself.

Instead of her name, she greeted with "Are you always so fired up? Sex with you must be a whirlwind."

Befriending silence on a dime, I knew neither how nor attained the sparkling wit to respond to her extrasensory, brusquely intimate introduction. Only now does it make me hoot with humble acknowledgment. Yes! It is always the two-minute warning at a tied Super Bowl. Let's do this! And touchdown.

"Whew," she said, "your energy. I'm exhausted. Aren't you exhausted? I know exactly where to start with you."

I sang nary a note. But the breathing and diaphragmatic relaxation techniques she started me out with were, and still are, as fundamental to any voice as they are to life.

I have been impatient all my life.

I have been impatient all my life.

I have been impatient all my life.

Like rehearsing and writing "I will raise my hand before shouting out the answer" on the chalkboard twenty times per teacher's instruction until it seeped into my brain, we have covered the fact that I am a slow learner. More accurately, I am a slow learner of things I do not want to hear.

Had the induction, the cesarean, the complications thereof, taught me nothing?

I couldn't wait—only to miscarry.

I could sit here and cry about it—the miscarriage, the impatience, the pattern—all over again.

Instead let me be grateful for what it…for what the one we lost… taught me.

For what it taught the stunted ten-year-old in me, the one who would rather control emotion than to feel it, the one who would rather act than to listen, the one who would rather cling to ego thinking a lot of herself because her father didn't, the child in me rebelling against the child in him.

My father was a complicated man, an intricate web of charming and talented and accessible intertwined with madness and destruction and impossible. He never knew an innocent childhood. His mother "hated" him and told him so, stealing any wholesomeness he may have had. She abused him, and he fed into the cycle and abused himself. A borderline and functioning alcoholic, quite possibly a borderline personality, diagnosed with PTSD as a drafted veteran of the Vietnam War, he wouldn't or couldn't admit that he needed help. He would rather deny, deny, deny. Of course, he didn't stop at himself. He took all of that injury and ire and stunted emotional growth and, at times, slung it at those nearest to him, at those who loved him most.

I always have to add "at times." He wasn't unbearable all the time. He could be decent. He was decent, at times. Maybe it makes me feel less a victim. I am not a victim; I never was.

And there it is…that chip, hoisting its defensive self upon my shoulder, jockeying for position against the ol' nag who doesn't yell everything. Even the chip is smart enough not to challenge the ol' battle-ax who does!

I did not have any control over the dysfunction—the hot mess—that was my family life as a child. But I did have control over how I would allow it to affect me. Boy, did I run with that. I did not *accept* my father's behavior, no more than he was willing to give acceptance to anyone else. It was wrong. He knew it. I knew it. Everyone in my household knew it. Although no one confronted him with that fact for a very long time. I would not *surrender* to my father's behavior. He would not break me. I was stronger than he. Even though I desperately wished he would give me reason to, I absolutely positively could not *trust* my father. I would have been a moron to do so. He—his mouth, his words, his favorite weapon—was going to be mean and nasty and hurtful…at times.

And at times, tit for tat, I got the hang of detachment, my heart growing impermeable as a castle. Moat, spiral staircase, talus, arrow slits, bent entrance, and trou-de-loup in place!

What I failed to realize was I had become so accustomed to being in control, so accustomed to forfeiting soft for hard, humility for strength, femininity for masculinity, that it became habitual, part of who I was or who I am.

Control, do, act—all steps my father would not take in any type of recovery, in any type of responsibility, in any type of healthy choice for himself…his family. Well, I had a choice, by God. Ugh, my attitude. Control, do, act—the trio represented to me initiative. Yes, I identified with all of that. And when did I want to initiate all of that? Yep, now.

What I failed to realize was one need not always lead with that boot. Sometimes controlling, doing, acting are merely Hail Marys, temporary solutions, refusals to look within…to *listen*. To *be*. To slow down long enough—*be patient*—to hear feeling, faith and instinct.

What I couldn't have known is to be vulnerable—susceptible to and reliant on one's own feeling, faith and instinct—*is* achieving, doing, on a completely different level. Empowerment without strategy, strength, exertion? Preservation without defense, protection, resistance? Impossible.

While vulnerable, I am my most courageous, my most powerful. I am so much more than I ever thought I could be.

I was vulnerable in my first birth. Yet the concept of vulnerability was something so foreign to me—something a ten-year-old girl promised herself she could outwit, outrun, outpower—I couldn't even identify it, flow with it, use it to my advantage…then.

The fear, the pep talks between contractions, the wanting to do it "right"—it was all misguided vulnerability. It was all about the future, thoroughly snubbing *the moment*. It was all about acting, doing, controlling, escaping powerlessness…when that is exactly how I ended up birthing, powerless amidst all the interventions.

What I couldn't have known is my uterus, my womb, my femaleness…*she* would be able to transform my life. The thing my father used to ridicule me for, the thing I tried desperately to compensate for—being female—would be my greatest virtue. Literally baby girl, figuratively me, earth mother, caregiver, woman, birth, miscarriage…*she* was about to storm the castle.

"There is no other organ quite like the uterus. If men had such an organ they would brag about it. So should we." —Ina May Gaskin

# No Outlet

*Your body knows how to do this. Your body knows how to do this. Your body knows how to do this.*

I chanted Genevieve's advice, the midfoot of each alternating foot running in 4/4 time on the pavement. Three to five miles at a time and often throughout my miscarriage, I ran until I no longer had to chant. Until the chant became embedded in my bones, as reactionary as my old brain.

I don't know that Genevieve would have approved. I wasn't necessarily taking it easy. But I *was* doing what came naturally to me. And it worked.

I canceled the ob-gyn appointment, committed to patience, committed to myself...committed to my body.

My body knew better than I exactly what I needed. My miscarriage took forever because I needed it to in order to heal...emotionally.

Optimism can propel me onward and upward before I am ready. Confidently negotiating emotion as though it were an obstacle course only to sprint across the finish line and realize I have accomplished nothing. The hurt remains. It lingers in my head and in my heart, with the patience of a monk, until I stomach it.

Accepting the miscarriage, surrendering to it, and trusting my body could handle it were essential.

Trust. Surrender. Accept. These are the recurring themes of my childbearing journey, the recurring themes of my motherhood journey, the recurring life themes that only childbearing and motherhood could get through my blockhead.

And the way it all transpired could not have been more obscure to me at the time it was transpiring, yet could not have been more obvious to me by the time the learning was received.

The cascade of interventions tipped off by an unnecessary induction, further leading to an unnecessary cesarean and all of its unnecessary complications were all necessary in my committing—another very basic quality that often eluded me—to a position about the way in which I would choose to birth.

The redundancy of a controlling, doing, acting—medical, obstetrical, hospital—birth and recovery experience led me to personally discover that I found valuable a way to birth in which controlling, doing, acting (i.e. intervening) have no roles.

In essence, it would take everything to show me nothing was the answer.

Birthing and mothering Mila, extraordinary bird, had been working on me. The one we were losing only provided reinforcement. Together they were calling me into the now, where doing does not matter so much as surrendering to the moment, whether to lap up the enjoyment of it or simply having to go through it. They were imparting on me the importance of patience, where listening, stillness, acceptance supersede knowing, noise, reaction. They were proving to me that I cannot control everything, so I may as well trust that I—mind and body—can navigate the course without being at the helm.

It would take childbearing, child-rearing, and losing a child to heal/fix/right negative reactionary themes from my own childhood. I could replace *control, do, act* with *trust, surrender, accept* and be just fine. The bottom would not fall out. Dysfunction would not prevail. It could be something beneficial, something quite beautiful actually, not only for me but for those I share my life with.

It would take the shortcut of a hospital birth to show me that home birth was not such a long shot after all. The disruptive and superfluous bells and whistles of that hospital birth were responsible for my seeking a natural path through an eight-week-long miscarriage that ultimately equipped me to birth at home with nothing but the essentials.

Conceivably the longest eight weeks of my life, body and instinct tested me. Knowing impatience to be my worst quality, they asked, how bad do you want it?

To which I replied/chanted Genevieve's empowering advice: Your body knows how to do this. Your body knows how to do this. Your body knows how to do this.

I do not know that I could have or would have done it without Genevieve.

In her midwifery sphere, surely those seven words are as unassuming as they are ordinary. Surely I am not the first she bestowed them upon. Albeit, those seven words made a difference not only in my miscarriage and in my second birth but in my life in general. Giving those seven words a chance and in the fullness of time giving in to them, I'll be darned if feeling didn't outshine opinion.

What's that saying about "opinion" and how nothing stands in the way of progress more than it? I quite like Augustus William Hare's take, "The feeling is often the deeper truth, the opinion the more superficial one."

But what does one do when taught to rely on reason more than feeling? Whether that reason is based in fact or not. Little Jane falls down and bumps her knee. It does in fact hurt, and she feels like crying, so she does. Then someone attempts to reason with Little Jane, "Shh, honey, don't cry. Look, there's no blood. You're okay. It's not that bad." The more developed and socialized and reasonable we grow, the more technologically advanced we become, the harder it is to find feeling—instinct—isn't it?

I *feel* like this can't be right. The sign says NO OUTLET. But the GPS says this is the way to go!

Somewhere over the course of those long-lived eight weeks, I finally gave in to faith and feeling, something other than detachment and opinion.

Neither belief nor bargain could stop what was happening. Nowhere to run, where could I run that the miscarrying uterus would not follow? NO OUTLET—damn GPS!

I was forced to shut up, shut it down, and listen. Be still and listen...not to me, the ego, I, the part of one's self under direct influence of the external world, the one bogged down in all the opinions. Listen inwardly. Close thine eyes and listen—heartbeat, breath, pulse, blood, bones, body, soul...instinct.

And there she was.

And her three-point plan was so simple in theory: Do nothing. Endure. Survive.

I wondered, maybe I just have the survival instincts of a sloth. It doesn't even make sense: survive by doing nothing?

Finding and following instinct is how I would come to learn that doing nothing *is* the hardest work of all.

# Egg Whites & BBT

SURRENDER. TRUST. ACCEPT. HUMILITY. FEEL. PAUSE. THIS PARENTING THING was shaking up the entire paradigm of my life.

I must have thought a hundred times, as I kissed Mila good night, how content I was. How I had never felt this inherently at peace before. I must have shown it a hundred vulnerable times, a few runaway tears spilling over blushing cheeks, as my head hit the pillow beside Wade's and I would say, "I don't know why I'm crying. I just never thought it could be like this."

I must have chalked it up to postpartum hormones a hundred times, too, when I woke the next morning and coached myself not to get lazy in my contentment. Continue to want, desire, achieve. Motherhood does not have to change your goals, your dreams, your life.

But it *was* changing my priorities and perspectives. Our miscarriage, distressing as it was, only helped me realize that, giving rise to new quotes and mantras:

"Be still, and know that I am God." —Psalm 46:10

"Slow down and everything you are chasing will come around and catch you." —John De Paola

"Thank everyone who calls out your faults, your anger, your impatience, your egotism; do this consciously, voluntarily." —Jean Toomer

"When you rise in the morning, give thanks for the light, your life, your strength. Give thanks for your food and for the joy of living." —Tecumseh

"To be content doesn't mean you don't desire more, it means you're thankful for what you have and patient for what's to come." —Tony Gaskins

I made a conscious effort to distance myself from obsession as best I could. Strange, I never considered myself "obsessive." Hardworking and persistent maybe, but not obsessive because I always associated obsession with someone, a person, a mate. I am not even obsessive about Wade, *the* love of my life. Before kids he had his life and I had mine. It is a wonder how exactly we came together, each quite adept at being alone and each quite covetous of such "me time."

Admission being the first step, I had to admit that I can be obsessive about undertaking things, about undertaking things that matter an awful lot to me. Like a dog with a wound, I will not leave it alone.

This whole having-another-child thing consumed a substantial portion of my thoughts and energy and motivation for nearly a year...only to miscarry. Push, force, do, obtain, make it happen...only to watch it dissolve without being able to *do* a damn thing about it.

So I stopped obsessing. I threw out the OPKs. I threw out the fertility calendar. I threw caution to the wind and made love to my beautiful man without scheduling it, neurotically around ovulation, of course.

And it felt good. Not the giving up part so much as the spontaneity. I was always quite spontaneous. Had I lost that in my recently acquired managerial role as mother, wife, coordinator of all things planned and structured?

The only thing I kept doing fertility-wise was tracking BBT—basal body temperature—and cervical mucus. Now this stuff, I could not stop. Who would want to? It is fascinating! An anatomy and science project all in one, I was getting pretty good at deciphering my body's— the body that knows a hell of a lot more than I do—ovulatory cues.

How could I have gone nearly forty years without so much as an inkling about "fertility awareness"? Practical knowledge, likely inherent or commonsensical at some point in history before birth control was widely available, that could help me in natural family planning.

Furthermore, how was it that the signs of natural family planning were staring me right in the face, yet I didn't even have the fertility awareness to recognize them?

I recall sitting in the office of the ob-gyn I consulted with when conception the second time around seemed out of reach. I failed to mention to her the scant and intermittent egg-white looking discharge I was experiencing every few weeks for fear the admission would result in some sort of prescription: antibiotic prescription to be precise. It was unfair of me to assume that her treatment would involve antibiotics at all, but I could not take the chance, as that lesson learned the hard way still scarred.

I did not inherently feel as though anything was wrong. It certainly did not present as anything that needed treatment. It didn't even seem like "discharge" as much as something that made my toilet paper slick from time to time. Reminiscent of losing my mucus plug with Mila, minus the blood tinge and much smaller in amount, I had never experienced anything like it before. Why would I, I guess, having been on birth control—which suppresses ovulation—most of my adult life.

I did, however, mention it to the nurse practitioner who worked with the ob-gyn and who took over where the ob-gyn left off in setting up my "fertility bloodwork." The NP and I hit it off instantly, mulling over an integrative approach to fertility. Her comments of my focusing not on conception but on overall health and well-being won my trust. By the time she mentioned acupuncture, massage, and yoga, I felt safe sharing with her lock, stock, and barrel.

"Egg white," the NP said, "well, are you ovulating?" As if anyone would or should know if they are.

I shrugged amidst answering, "I'm going to start using the predictor sticks."

Maybe it was the shrug or obvious lack of fertility lingo—"predictor sticks"—that led her to perform a prompt vaginal swab before excusing herself to wherever a microscope and a slide resided. How exciting! Action, and root cause analysis, rather than prescription.

Within minutes, she returned. "Normal cervical fluid." To which she tied in a gripping tutorial on cervical fluid/mucus and how it changes with one's menstrual cycle.

My *bothersome* and intermittent "egg whites" were nature's cue—my body's cue—a telltale sign from my cervix that I was entering and/

or in the midst of my "fertile window," about to ovulate. Duh!

Off I went, armed with information, which always turns into obsession for me—for more information and then of course application of more information—somehow, fortunately, unfortunately.

Cervical fluid, cervical position, OPKs, BBT: you name it, I tracked it. A regular virtuoso at timing intercourse with ovulation, I found great fulfillment in feeling in sync with my body, my reproductive cues.

But ultimately it didn't matter.

Conception was not something I could control. Even after seemingly willing it into existence with another pregnancy, conception was not something I could learn enough about to maintain. The only definitive thing I learned about conception is that it is miraculous, truly mystifying.

So in my bid to stop obsessing, I finally committed to giving up tracking BBT and cervical mucous, too. I was on my last BBT charting sheet. Having stockpiled them initially, this would be it. Done. Zero. Zilch. Nada. But I couldn't stop now. Another annoying compulsion, I *have* to finish anything I start.

Is it just me, or is it universally a rare thing for the universe to be on schedule?

Or is it my timing that is off. Or maybe the universe thinks, for some reason, I need the shock and awe. But the things I think I want the most at any given time are not the things that are meant for me at that time. Then the things I learn not to want are the things that are meant for me, but only once I go through the steps of not wanting them.

To top it off, these things have to come in some dramatic fashion that is either soul-soaring or crow-eating or tongue-in-cheek. Case in point: When the universe welcomed me at my birth, just as I was crowning all of the lights went out. No storm, no blanket power outage, a blackout limited to the hospital, no lie. Yes, I was literally "born in the dark."

I spent half a year, post-miscarriage, convincing myself that parents to a singleton we would be. Mila was it, more than enough. How could we ever love another child the way we love her? We would have

more of everything to give to her. More love, more time, more expend-
able income for any and all of her interests. We wouldn't have to split
ourselves between two children, maybe even lending itself to some of
that long gone but longed for "me time" for mama and daddy.

Of course I blogged and shared a post on Facebook about it, seeking support and direction from singletons and parents of singletons.

And...

*Boom!* went the universe.

Color me stupefied morning after morning, and over the course of
two weeks, when my final BBT chart produced the textbook phantom-
esque "triphasic pattern." Astonishingly after what I thought to be
ovulation, guesstimating by my old friend egg white cervical mucus,
my basal body temperature spiked and spiked and spiked again.

I remained unexcitable, as I had read the pattern could be misleading. Rare on most any chart, the quintessential triphasic pattern might
show up in twelve percent of cases. And in that twelve percent, it does
not necessarily equate to pregnancy.

Nearly one month to the day that I went public with my "singleton" blog and Facebook post, I would have my last menstrual period. In
the sparse twelve percent, I tripped over my jaw for days. My triphasic
BBT equated to pregnancy?

Yes...

It did.

Oh...

You whimsical little universe.

Yes...

I was chock-full of crow. Indeed, my soul wanted to soar.

But...

It did not dare.

# Hurry Up And Wait

Birth is a lot like film—hard work and an art.

Any witness to the last minutes of birth and any witness to the final cut of a movie could easily overlook all of the behind-the-scenes hours of hard work it took to get there.

Much like my assumption that dabbling in film would be glamorous, I would discover that pregnancy and birth are not glamorous either. One of the most unglamorous elements of both to this impatient individual was all of the hurrying to wait.

My first birth—certainly to include prenatal visits—was a series, and a rude awakening, of hurry up and wait. I don't know why I was put out by the hurrying to wait, as that grind seems to be the standard in our healthcare system. Maybe I assumed that since I felt so unique in my pregnant body, carrying new life, that I would be treated differently…uniquely.

Imagine, then, the pleasant surprise when in my prenatal visits with Genevieve, my time was as valued as her time. Each allotted hour at each prenatal visit was actually spent with her and was indeed productive. Continuity of care was never broken. Every time we had an appointment, we saw Genevieve. Any and all care, to include routine assessments and bloodwork, was provided by Genevieve. She has a lovely apprentice, Katie, who took part as well.

For the hour spent in Genevieve's office, fifteen minutes may have been allocated to assessment. The rest of the time was spent talking, educating, informing. Amazing! I showed up with a list of questions and she answered them—with additional pointers at every turn—patiently repeating herself as I had many repetitive questions. Part sage and part counselor, she informed and encouraged me through my apprehension, committed to helping me prepare and navigate through the labor and birth I desired.

"Communal" comes to mind. Not only did she educate in her office at private appointments, she offered and encouraged clients to partake in complimentary group birthing classes. In these classes, I found a certain nurture and warmth in being around other pregnant women. Wade found camaraderie and relief in being around other birth partners who shared many of the same concerns and fears that he had. Mila found a few new friends, as the classes were a family affair, with the supplementary topic of "sibling preparation" for the newborn's arrival.

This approach allowed me to feel a part of a midwifery and home-birther community, a part of something larger than just my pregnancy. Maybe this is the way I envision past generations of women experiencing pregnancy and birth when cocooned in the wisdom and support of other women. Much like the birth I aimed for, it felt natural.

Right off, I learned that midwives attend. "I have attended two hundred births." That was Genevieve's verb of choice: "attend." She did not deliver babies. Birthing women delivered babies. She did not attend deliveries. She attended births.

I vividly recall it being so striking and purposeful in comparison to how I had heard most healthcare providers refer to birth—"vaginal delivery," "cesarean delivery," "I deliver one hundred babies a year." Genevieve didn't have to explain it, and I didn't have to ask. It was in the way she purposely chose her words, in the way she said it, as though she may be informing me of something I had never heard before. And I hadn't.

What a perspective. Birthing women and their babies are not delivered but attended. She who grows and nourishes and carries her child births it, regardless of how exactly that birth transpires. It is her body that delivers—surrenders—the child. Birth belongs to birthing women, and their partners.

Similarly, prenatal care belongs to pregnant women. Routine tests offered under Genevieve's care were roughly the same in amount as what I experienced with prenatal care in my first pregnancy. The remarkable thing was that I had an active role in cherry-picking tests and/ or treatments that made the best and safest sense to me. A cornerstone of the midwifery model of care is that pregnant and birthing women's choices are foremost and should be supported as safely as possible.

For instance, Genevieve's standard was to offer one ultrasound, the twenty-week anatomy ultrasound. She made clear to me that if I felt the ultrasound unwarranted, I did not have to accept it at all. When I in fact requested an ultrasound, in addition to and before the anatomy scan, at thirteen weeks—needing to see for myself that this child was with me, hear for myself that this child had a heartbeat—she set that up for me immediately.

When I vocalized concern about weekly cervical exams from week thirty-six and beyond, Genevieve informed me that they were not a part of her standard but should I change my mind and request any, she would certainly oblige.

I appreciated the choices. It was empowering and fulfilling to know that my choices mattered, that my choices would shape my pregnancy and birth experience.

I found Genevieve's natural approach in treating "all the livelong damn day sickness" with nutrition particularly helpful and comforting in not having to worry with prescriptions. In my first pregnancy when I sought natural remedies for persistent first-trimester nausea, I was prescribed medication. Medication that seemed to me unnecessary, and only left me to wonder was I being irresponsible in not taking it.

The practical advice Genevieve gave in stressing the importance of eating every few hours to ward off/contain nausea seemed not only sound to me but was effective. Even if only a handful, she said, be sure not to skimp on protein. In the handy-dandy "client information packet" given to me upon my first official prenatal visit, she volunteered nutrition information as it pertained to pregnancy. "The protein counter" was especially useful in meeting daily quotas. And "herbal allies" was a cool and informative addition that brought to my awareness an entirely new and natural world of herbs beneficial not only to abating pregnancy-induced symptoms, such as nausea, but herbs that actually support pregnancy and even health beyond pregnancy.

A nice detail about home birth was that Genevieve came to us for a visit/appointment once we reached full-term. This allowed her to familiarize herself with our home and at least get a bird's eye view before birth was upon us. Another in-home appointment was scheduled with a partnering midwife who would also attend our birth, as Genevieve preplans to have two midwives—herself included—present at every home birth from transition on.

Those home visits were like walking into the gym and finding that the Smith machine is free. At full-term, the least amount of time spent behind a steering wheel made this expectant mama pretty dang happy. The home visits also provided a nice segue into staying home and having them come to us for the birth. Again, it felt only natural that the last weeks of pregnancy were spent at home where we would birth, and where Genevieve would return to us periodically over the next few weeks for follow-up appointments.

It is no accident that women have, on average, forty weeks of gestation. I needed forty weeks to prepare.

Whether it was her reading list, her group classes, her one-on-one tutoring, her promotion of not only physical but mental and spiritual health of pregnancy and childbirth, Genevieve fostered my preparation. Visualize labor and birth from beginning to end to include even the birth of the placenta, she advised. Imagine it all, in various ways should one's reality veer from ideal. Set the course for doing it all.

Carefully covering all bases from conceptual to tangible, hands down the most captivating thing to me in Genevieve's treasure trove of midwifery traditions was abdominal palpation.

Upon the bump growing to a palpable size—somewhere around the twentieth week—Genevieve palpated my abdomen at each prenatal appointment to assess baby's position. Exciting and educational, nothing if not preparatory, too, I found great purpose and joy in it. It was the thing I most looked forward to at each appointment. With my hands beneath my midwife's, an otherwise obscured baby was literally made tangible. Genevieve led me on a guided discovery—head, backbone, bottom. That's a baby. Right there. Beneath my hands. *My* baby.

Could I later discover those same parts? Um, no. But at each successive appointment, my midwife who had honed this time-honored midwifery skill would enlighten me. As a rule, baby was in LOA or ROA position—left occiput anterior or right occiput anterior. These terms became quite familiar to me while under midwifery care. These terms are more than just terms. These terms are knowledge, awareness.

Concretely feeling baby aided in actualizing a sweet nugget of growing flesh and bones in my uterus. By the time labor rolled around, visualizing baby's position was second nature to me, which was helpful in envisioning what was happening in utero with contractions and descent and flexion and rotation and crowning and ultimately birth. I did not have to go an entire pregnancy without knowing I was carrying a child in the most disadvantageous position for delivery, the way I did with baby girl.

Like the morning I woke and inherently felt something had changed with baby's position. If memory serves correctly, I was in my twenty-sixth week. Up to that point, I had been so uncomfortable in how I was carrying. My abs hurt, my bladder hurt, my skin hurt. Everything felt stretched to the limit. Except for this particular morning. Though subtle, the shape of my abdomen had actually changed. No longer round and full from diaphragm to pubic bone, it felt kind of deflated at the top. I could inhale completely, filling my lungs without resistance. Everything felt too good, too similar to my pregnancy with baby girl who I carried posteriorly without the slightest clue.

"Okay, so baby's changed position on us," Genevieve confirmed instinct, double-checking with palpating hands.

Once I moved from the daybed and back into the love seat, she began to address OP—occiput posterior—position.

"It's nothing to be particularly concerned about at this point. Some babies are posterior up until and even through delivery. Many will turn on their own before crowning."

With a baby doll and a mock female bony pelvis, she provided an interactive tutorial on the seven cardinal movements of labor—engagement, descent, flexion, internal rotation, extension, external rotation, and expulsion.

Then, she went on to explain what I could do to help baby get back into and stay in anterior position. Modern furniture no friend to the OP positioned babe, I would learn that my position had a lot to do with baby's. Rather than sit at my desk in a chair, I could sit on a birthing ball to encourage good posture. Rather than recline on my back, I could adopt left-side lying position with a pillow between my knees. Rather than perpetually sit on my bum, I could take intermittent breaks from sitting for long periods of time. I could get on my hands and knees, or at the very least on my knees with my elbows propped upon a couch and leaning forward, a few times a day for fifteen to twenty minutes at a time.

If I wanted to nix furniture altogether and rely on my body to seat itself, I could spend as much time as I could stand in resting squat position. And if I had a mind to, I could seek prenatal chiropractic care or prenatal bodywork. Not only bringing relief to a pregnant body, these types of activities can encourage strong and supple pelvic muscles, which in turn can encourage optimal fetal position.

Basically I could think of my pregnant belly as a "hammock" and my spine as a "tree." Any movement I made or any position I was in, I could attempt to maneuver myself in such a way that baby's back and bottom would fancy the hammock rather than the tree.

"You could even try putting a heating pad on your abdomen to draw baby's back there. Babies are drawn to warmth," Genevieve offered one more "could do."

And the light bulb went off! I had been using a heating pad on my lower back for general pregnancy-induced aches since my last visit. A heating pad that I laid on my bed and then lied on flat on my back.

"Oh, don't stop using the heating pad," she advised when I confessed. "If it helps, use it. Just bring it around your abdomen, too. Lie on your side on the heating pad, wrapping half of it around your back and the other half around your abdomen. Or you could sit back on the heating pad for a spell. Just be sure to put a pillow or something behind your lumbar to support the natural curve there, supporting baby's position."

She stressed not to worry about positioning. Just relax and take care of your homework (i.e. daily anterior-position-persuading exercises). Maybe even use it as meditation. Visualize baby in anterior position.

Visualize baby descending into the pelvis, as she showed me on the model. Visualize it daily. And if I feel "wiggles" or "tickles" in my lower abdomen, right above my pubic bone, that is likely baby's fingers—a strong indicator that baby is in OP position.

"No waaay," I exhausted with an enamored smile. "That happened just this morning." I totally felt the pubic bone tickles! I remember thinking, Hmm…that's new. New to this pregnancy, but common with baby girl.

How did she know this? All of this? This woman, this midwife, was so smart, intuitive, commonsensical. At every prenatal visit, she was going to give me a tidbit that would be useful in my preparation. She just was…going to…every single time.

And every time, my mind would go back to my first pregnancy and wonder why I could not recall any tidbits…if ever I received any.

I could go on and on about the differences, from the obvious to the microscopic, in how our first and likely our last pregnancy and labor and birth were managed. Evidence-based information and evidence-based practice, preparation, choice, faith in the natural process, and faith in myself and my body were paramount differences.

There was no preconception, no pressure, no hurry up and wait.

There was no "We can give it a try." The new motto was a devoted "Your body knows how to do this." No doubt, those seven words still flood my confidence cup.

Again, I quote Robbie Davis-Floyd, "I have long believed and have stated many times in my oral presentations that the most important determinants of the outcome of a woman's birth are the attitudes and ideology of her primary caregiver(s)."

# Expecting

I WOULD GO AN ENTIRE PREGNANCY BEFORE FULLY BELIEVING NATURAL LABOR and birth would—could—be my thing.

To this day I marvel at our little man and think, wow, you're really here.

I just had that specific thought while peeking in on his celestial sleeping self. My heart. Sleeping babies make that four-chambered, blood-pumping, life-sustaining organ leap right up into the back of your throat, don't they. It is an instant catch...bittersweet...conflicted between feelings of joy and longing. Joy for such a treasure, joy that the treasure is healthy and thriving, all the while understanding the very flourishing of the treasure causes the longing. It is impossible to go back and live and feel and breathe that sweetness of new life again. That first year—all of them, really—is so ephemeral.

What is that saying about the rearview mirror? It is smaller than the windshield because what's behind us is not as important as what's in front of us.

Fantastic premise, but certainly whoever came up with it was never affected by miscarriage. It was nearly impossible to keep from looking over my shoulder, wondering if the past would repeat itself.

I remember first spotting. Mila and I had just returned from a run at Town Lake. I remember the morning of the ultrasound. Mila had Gymboree prior to our appointment where we stopped off at Gateway Shopping Center and window-shopped before stores or Gymboree even opened. I was so unsettled about the appointment that we had been up and ready for hours.

I remember a wedding we attended at the end of May when we were thrilled that my period was recently MIA. I remember a wedding we attended at the end of July when we were actively miscarrying, celebrating and smiling and putting up a good front.

I remember a night when after bath and books bedtime ritual, seven-thirty on the dot, Mila was having a hard time staying asleep. This was unusual for her, a lover of routine. I had just come from the bathroom, after one of those intermittent and gut-wrenching gushes. I cried out for her as much as she cried out for me. Holding her and holding back tears, we rocked and lamented. It was as if she knew something was askew, though she knew not what exactly.

People, events, clothing I wore, places—as insignificant as gas stations—were, and foreseeably will always be, tethered to that miscarriage.

It was anchored in my psyche until baby boy was born at thirty-eight weeks and six days. An atonement of sorts?

Until then I tried desperately to have no expectations.

No easy feat for a woman who is expecting.

It never dawned on me how correct that term is when referring to pregnancy. "We're expecting...," "She's expecting...," "They're expecting...a baby."

For the longest time it seemed redundant. Of course they're expecting a baby. What else would they have? A velociraptor?

But *expecting*—regard something as likely to happen—is perfect. It is probable and promising, but not promised.

The pre-miscarriage me would have been inspired by inventor Charles Kettering, "High achievement always takes place in the framework of high expectation."

The post-miscarriage me went with philosopher Lao Tzu, "Act without expectation."

I still can't quite wrap my mind around how it came to be that a miscarriage actually prepared me better than anything else could have for pregnancy, labor, and birth. It is uncanny. But it did. Expect nothing. Be present.

Mila schooled me, too.

Staying home with her, I had become accustomed to the reclusiveness that engenders, which was no abrupt adjustment seeing how writing is a rather solitary activity. Taking her lead, my world became very small yet grand at the same time. And she kept me honest.

"I'm Spirit and you're Rain, Mama," Mila set the scene from her favorite movie *Spirit: Stallion of the Cimarron*.

"Yes, baby, I'm Rain," I replied, already failing my "be present" test. The pencil in my hand did not stop multitasking, sketching a music video storyboard and making a grocery list, whilst I juggled committing to play with my lovely.

"No, Mama, get into it," she demanded. "Like this..." A series of whinnies and neighs, convincing and very horse-like, escaped her, her head vigorously shaking about a mess of blonde hair—her mane, of course. "We're wild and free." A premise of the movie, Spirit is an untamable Mustang of the Old West. "Come on, Mama, you have to be wild and free!"

To which I finally put down my pencil, vaulted out of my chair and kicked up my *hooves*, galloping after her down the hallway. "Neighhhhhhh!" And you know what? That grocery list could not have cared less that it was not done.

Our first and the one we lost would be the Zen masters.

This time I *could* wait.

Replacing impatience with gratitude and expectation with humility, for every morning that I woke and still a life thrived inside of me, I was thankful.

I told myself I wasn't going to get attached to the bud in my belly until it actually sprouted. Yeah, that went well...

Something a bit more attainable, I opted for a low profile instead, which only made easier my attempts to slowly and deliberately live in the moment. Tuning out the excess, committing to doing less by leaving breathing room in my schedule so that I could be mindfully into whatever I was doing without thinking about all there was yet to be done, innately shifted my point of view. I even discovered that my daily cooking ritual did not have to be mundane, a chore; it could serve generously not only my family but as an exercise in meditation, being present. I began to feel very much like one of those "private pregnant women" Ruth Morgan poetically summed up:

"Pregnant women! They had that weird frisson, an aura of magic that combined awkwardly with an earthy sense of duty. Mundane, because they were nothing unique on the suburban streets; ethereal because their attention was ever somewhere else. Whatever you said was trivial. And they had that preciousness which they imposed wherever they went, compelling attention, constantly reminding you that they carried the future inside, its contours already drawn, but veiled, private, an inner secret."

An exercise in courage, I did go public with a blog somewhere around the twenty-week mark.

Whatever it—our pregnancy—would or would not be, I wanted to acknowledge it, honor it. I had a bit of angst in doing so. Was I going to jinx it? I knew, and knew of, women who miscarried and/or experienced stillbirths at or well after twenty weeks. I knew, and knew of, women whose membranes ruptured prematurely at twenty weeks or thirty weeks, where babies fought for their first weeks and months of life in NICUs. There were so many things that could go wrong.

Stop! How is this—worrying—living in the moment? Post the damn blog already.

You are pregnant…right now…in this moment. *Just be*…pregnant.

And there were some iffy—test of faith—things that happened throughout this pregnancy versus the "unremarkable" first one.

As conception took hold and all the livelong damn day sickness gave me hope by coming on like gangbusters, Mila came down with a monster tummy bug. The child had never been sick before, barely even a runny nose. How convenient she would catch something while we were in our crucial first trimester where miscarriage is most common, and while we were traveling, no less. Over the clouds and puking on a plane, to grandmother's house we go!

Of course I caught it, too. I couldn't tell you the last time I had a stomach bug, but there was no mistaking I had it then…eight weeks into a pregnancy already teeming with nausea, and on the distant heels of a miscarriage.

That's how it's gonna be, huh! Shoulder nag who yells everything shouted into the darkness of my mother's guest bedroom where I lie beneath a heap of blankets shivering yet burning up at the same time. Fever in early pregnancy cannot be good! Why now! You're gonna test me every step of the way, huh!

Oh, no one's testing you. Calm down, drama queen. Shoulder nag who doesn't yell everything interjected. You're not that feverish. It's going to break and then it will be over.

"...how it's gonna *be*, huh!" "...it will *be* over." Both nags' assertions recommitted me to "act without expectation." It is going to be what it is going to be, so—just *be*.

I had already told Genevieve, casually informing her via email that I suspected we were preggers and that I would be in touch if and when we made it to the ten-week mark, as she would want to schedule our first prenatal visit at that point. In my best blasé tone, my email read, "Hey, there, my period is MIA. But it has only been six weeks since my LMP. We're going on vacay for a few weeks. If we're still pregnant when we return, I'll be in touch."

So I breathed...in and out until I felt relaxed in my bones...underneath that heap of blankets. Mila sleeping soundly beside me and without vomitus for an entire day, I cuddled around her, grateful the worst was over for her. And to the child in my womb, hold on in there, I sent the encouraging thought. It's up to you, I continued, confused if I was talking to baby or God, surely a bit of both. Regardless of what exactly the *be* would be, I topped it off by chanting Wade's laidback anthem: *Everything's gonna be alright. Everything's gonna be alright. Everything's gonna be alright.*

Growing up on the East Coast and with swiftness in my blood, I wonder if it is a prerequisite for homegrown Texans, or maybe just Austinites, to be so cool—laid back.

Maybe I have been here long enough that they are rubbing off on me. Maybe that is why I did not lose it when sometime in my late second/early third trimester, and on only one occasion, I got up from the potty and bright red blood was mixed in with my urine. We had just returned from Mila's Saturday morning Soccer Shots.

"Oh, shit," I said, surprisingly matter-of-fact. "Hmm…well, that's not so good."

"What?" Wade inquired, within earshot.

"I have, ah…a little blood in my urine?" I questioned what I hoped to be the lesser concern. Better to be coming from the urinary tract than the uterus, right?

"Did that ever happen with Mila?"

"Nope."

"Well, shouldn't we go to the hospital, or something?"

"No. No, we shouldn't," I replied. "Let me call Genevieve." The one who has faith in my body, the one who has faith in this process.

Hell to the yeah-sss! Shoulder nag who yells everything chimed in, pleased as punch that I was listening to and giving instinct a chance.

Inherently, I did not feel like anything was wrong. I felt fine. No cramping, no pain, no fever, no mucus (i.e. mucus plug), no dribbling of water, nothing other than the disconcerting blood, which was scant. And after talking with Genevieve, I felt even better. She asked some questions, ruling out an emergency situation, then explained how the cervix and its blood flow can change during pregnancy, sometimes manifesting as spotting/bleeding. She had me swing by for a urine culture in case of a UTI, which yielded negative results. Further instructing I pay close attention to all bathroom trips, notifying her of any more spotting/bleeding. She checked in with me that night and the next morning. On a Saturday night and a Sunday morning, no less, "after hours" in any other obstetrical world.

It proved to be nothing significant, one random precarious potty episode, thankfully.

Have you ever wondered why the wolf knocks on *three* little pigs' doors or why Goldilocks tastes *three* bears' porridge, or why there are not two or four but *three* musketeers?

Omne trium perfectum—"rule of three"—is a writing principle that suggests "events or characters introduced in threes are more humorous, satisfying, or effective in execution of the story and engaging the reader."

Assuming any of that is true, maybe the universe thought itself engaging in fulfilling the rule of three. Yes, there was one more incident aside from the Ugh Bug and the Spotty Potty. In an attempt not to be crude, we'll just call it Micturating Myself.

Hopefully it is "effective" because I found it neither "humorous" nor "satisfying" at the time.

I had read to Mila and tucked her in for a nap. Who am I kidding, it had become my nap, too, coveting the luxury in this pregnancy. Curiously enough, I could not sleep. We were well into the third trimester, and discomfort in the form of growing pains was setting in. I slipped out of bed so as not to rouse with my restlessness the cherub—aka personal sleeping furnace—curled up at my back.

I felt like I could pee. When couldn't I these days? I just went before lying down with Mila. Pride, for whatever asinine reason, took issue with this peeing business and bypassed the bathroom. Pick your battles! The ol' nag nagged. Peeing isn't one of them!

Oh, shut up, you, I dismissed. Doesn't she know I am tired. Of her opinion *and* yelling, I was unsure which exhausted me more.

My lower back feeling achy and pulled—lordotic—I dipped into resting squat position in the middle of the living room floor. This was something I did often throughout the day, and without incident, for the relief it brought in strengthening and lengthening.

No sooner than the backs of my thighs met the backs of my calves, she brayed again, I told you so!

Yep, I micturated myself.

But…I couldn't be certain that it wasn't amniotic fluid. So…I freaked out a bit.

"Oh, no, no, no, no, no, this is so not good," I talked nervously to myself, calculating the amount of weeks before term. "You're not ready, baby. There's plumping and CNS and brain and lungs…" Shit, shit, shit, shit, shit! I thought, unable to get the words out for the muffling lump sprinting its way up my esophagus. Blinking back tears, I tried to assess whatever fluid came out of wherever.

Clear.

Like that settles anything, urine *and* amniotic fluid can be clear!

Nose to carpet, I sniffed, to no avail. Lacking a canine's fire hydrant sense of smell, it smelled like nothing to me. Carpet, maybe?

Of course I called Genevieve, immediately feeling better after talking through it with her. Her hunch, the pressure on an already full bladder with the resting squat forced some urine out. But how could that be! I hadn't peed myself in…well, longer than I previously hadn't had a stomach bug.

I breathed. I listened to Genevieve. In turn, I listened to my body, instinct. I did not feel as though anything was wrong. And it wasn't. I kept track of baby's movements, looking for any change therein. I had no further leakage. Genevieve swung by the house the following morning—already in the area for a home visit to a fellow homebirther nearing her due date—for a litmus test that was negative for amniotic fluid. I am sure she gave the accommodation nary a second thought, but I did. In what other obstetrical world does the litmus paper make house calls.

I think about my water trickle with Mila and the onslaught of angst and haste thereafter. How it could have prevailed again, dependent on caregiver. I could have called a general number to reach a general person—nothing from the horse's mouth and clearly no home visit—who would have only alarmed me to come in immediately, consisting of waking Mila from her nap, or miss general office hours and go directly to a general ER. All for what—micturating myself?

I would say the rule of three *was* effective. It, like Mila, kept me honest. Those three unpredictable events, distributed over the pregnancy, kept it fresh how vulnerable pregnancy and time and life is in general. How important it was to be in the moment, to be thankful for the moment, to live and breathe in the moment. How important it was to remember we were promised nothing, only expecting.

# Chant Sheet

THE SUMMER BEFORE MY JUNIOR YEAR—AKA THE SUMMER THIS LATE BLOOMER'S boobs finally came in—Tina Turner's biographical film *What's Love Got to Do with It* finally released in theaters.

Taken with the scene that depicts the Queen of Rock 'n' Roll meditating and chanting "Nam Myoho Renge Kyo," I couldn't wait for some alone time to attempt it in the privacy of my bedroom. Not that my sixteen-year-old self got much out of it other than her curiosity quelled. My upbringing at the far end of Zen, nobody I knew meditated or chanted. If they did, they didn't tell me!

Turner's poignant and triumphant story of overcoming abuse at the hands of her then-husband Ike left an impression on me. I found fascinating the inference to meditation and chanting in helping her conquer and ultimately leave that dysfunction.

If meditation and chanting had that kind of power, impact, influence, how could I channel something like that in my own life?

I attempted it, in vain, many times: As a young adult, in my twenties, in my thirties, inside, outside, on the beach, in the snow, at sunrise, at sunset, in Sukhasana pose. "Nam Myoho Renge Kyo. Nam Myoho Renge Kyo. Nam Myoho Renge Kyo." No matter where or how or with whom I meditated or chanted, it did not seem to do much for me. I did not understand it. It did not resonate.

Until I miscarried.

Until I miscarried naturally. Until I did nothing and let my body do what it does. Until I got it through my thick skull that meditating and chanting is meant to do the opposite of doing.

In the childbirth preparation book *Birthing From Within*, chanting is described as a "self-hypnotic jingle."

A jingle? Now that was something the songwriter in me could relate to.

"Self-hypnotic jingle" pertains to a self "hope," "a particular behavior, belief, or outcome." One example used in *Birthing From Within* is from a lady named "Nikki," who made up her own self-hypnotic jingle: "I am a big, strong birthing machine."

Beats my first thought! In labor and in our first birth, pre-midwife and pre-preparation, all I could think was "I don't know what to do."

*Birthing From Within* simplified my comprehension of what chanting does to the brain and the body, why chanting works, essentially. "Repetition moves the new idea from your left brain to your right brain, and down into your body." "Rhythmic jingles that evoke vivid imagery activate your right brain and thus directly affect your body."

You mean, I don't just chant to chant? An attempt to find some third eye or center myself or bring about positivity or enlightenment or something? Chanting *is* practical?

My first success with chanting was not a conscious effort. I was not still. My eyes were not closed. My hands were not in any specific position—mudra.

I was running and simply saying to myself over and over again Genevieve's encouraging advice: *Your body knows how to do this.*

I did not know specifically that I was chanting. I only knew that I wanted and needed to believe her advice. So I simply kept repeating it, day after day and run after run, until I believed it. Until it actually worked.

Repetition. Repetition. "Repetition...is the mother of all learning."

How many of you when studying materials for exams, or for any other recall purpose, innately read the highlights, maybe even aloud, over and over again? Methodically, rhythmically—chanting, even if unwittingly—until comprehension forms, until you can readily pull from memory that which you need.

A, B, C, D, E, F, G...next time won't you sing with me. I would wager that we have all chanted to grasp concepts.

And how many of you study/read/chant while pacing or twirling a pencil or picking your nails or some other reflexive movement? According to some forward-thinking neuroscientists and educators alike, there is a reason for this: "The part of the brain that processes movement is the same part of the brain that processes learning."[1]

If a distant elementary school experience haunts you—"Sit still and pay attention," said many a teacher—there is a legitimate reason we were all a bunch of wiggle worms. Our instincts were most likely attempting to do what comes naturally to them, to establish the mind-body connection. Reasonably the best explanation as to why we were better able to concentrate and perform, better able to show restraint in keeping our derrières in chairs, *after* recess.

In aiming for wellness to include nourishment in the aftermath of my cesarean complications, I said to Wade, "Hey, babe, this 'ancestral eating' stuff sounds pretty legit. You wanna give it a try?"

"Sure," he said with a shrug. Then he chuckled distressingly before continuing, "Gonna be a rough twenty-one days."

That was his layman's equivalent to Aristotle's "It is frequent repetition that produces a natural tendency."

I gave myself a cushion. As opposed to twenty-one days, I banked on twenty-six weeks to shape my natural tendency where it came to labor and birth. Targeting the second and third trimesters, I applied frequent repetition in reading over and over again chants compiled from birth preparation books.

One birth preparation book in particular that I somehow stumbled upon in a "natural pregnancy book" search totally rocked my pregnant world. A book that made me an earnest student of birth, I feel forever indebted to its authors.

After all, it—peeking its sunshine yellow cover from the opening of my handbag—was how I surmised Genevieve would be a good match for me in our midwife-homebirther alliance.

Amidst introductions, and before I even knew that it was on her "client reading list," Genevieve pointed to the book and said, "I see you're reading *Birthing From Within*."

She knew about and even recommended this book? This book I was engrossed in. This book that spoke to me. Yes! Genevieve and I would do just fine. This book spoke of joy, mystery, preparation, self-discovery, awareness, surrender, natural pain management techniques, hard work, and compassion. This book represented the atmosphere in which I wanted to labor and birth. This book had me from page XII where it listed its number one of fifteen "philosophical assumptions and guiding principles of birthing from within childbirth classes":

1. Childbirth is a profound rite of passage, not a medical event (even when medical care is part of the birth).

It was the first time I, with a *medical* background, had heard it put that way. It was the first time I was exposed to that type of birth ideology. And I liked it. It resonated with me. Its stirring introduction ultimately drove me to explore what else I did not know but should know, be exposed to, about childbirth.

Bringing to mind an Alfred North Whitehead quote, "It requires a very unusual mind to undertake the analysis of the obvious."

On I embarked, analyzing it all…obscure and "obvious." My jaw gaping, my heart full with hope, my hands stingily clutched to books, I read about calm yet climactic, moving yet still, intuitive yet attended births. Births I never witnessed, let alone heard of, propelled and inspired me to keep reading until the obscure became the obvious—the norm.

From that analysis, I compiled a list—four standard letter-sized pages worth—of quotes, bullet points, principles that would become my preparation, my repetition, my chants.

Anything I read/analyzed was fair game to end up on my Chant Sheet. Yes, kind of like a "cheat sheet," it provided quick reference. However, for twenty-six weeks, I put that Chant Sheet to memory in my mind and in my body, putting Aristotle's "frequent repetition = natural tendency" theory to the test.

Every day, often multiple times a day and always at naptime, I recited my Chant Sheet. Always mandatory at naptime, lying in bed and drifting off to sleep and focusing on nothing but the bud in my belly. I loved this time. Just me and baby, Mila cuddled up to the bump and asleep beside us. So sweet. So fulfilling. But more than that, we were preparing. Not only chanting and believing myself, I was chanting to baby—This is how we are going to do it. We can do this, love.

The worse for wear, even stamped with the ubiquitous coffee stain, I still have my Chant Sheet. Reading over it from time to time, it always provides instant nostalgia and a good test of memory recall. I believe I will frame it sooner or later and hang it in the bedroom…over the bed… the one baby boy was made and born in.

If any one thing was key in my birth preparation, it was my Chant Sheet. Not only the acquainting myself with it but the compiling of it, too. Combing through tons of information and carefully selecting that which seemed foundational to me—that which made the final cut on the Chant Sheet—was most revealing, as the themes began to emerge:

The mind of the beginner is empty and open to all possibilities. The more ways you envision yourself giving birth, the more power you bring to your birth. Approach labor with an attitude of learning rather than control, an open-ended curiosity rather than a specific goal. *Forget all you think you know.* Trust instinct—the old brain, the primitive brain, the body brain, the one that knows without knowing. Birth in your body, not in your head. Just let it happen. *Your body knows how to do this.* Do not be afraid. Fear is about the future. Be in the moment. Labor has its own clock. It is N:OW (now o'clock). Every moment is N:OW. Pain is not static. Pain is temporary. I do not have to go through an entire labor! I can only experience *one* contraction, *one* rest, *one* push—in any moment. That *one* moment is always *now*. Pain is purposeful; stretch receptors, endorphins, dilation fuel labor. *Give in to it.* Struggle and fight, I sink. Relax, I float. Find the place within where my birth warrior lies. Go to the edge and beyond. Mind and ego melt to the background, inhibitions and trappings of our social selves are peeled away. The strength and power of labor is not demure; *the animal is there for all to see.* Into the destructive element, immerse myself. Be empty. Be open. Do nothing. Nothingness *is* naturalness. Do not think. Labor works best when you are out of your head. The less I *do*, the more nature will *do* for me. If you must *do* anything, *do surrender…*

# Pain Cube

Empty. Adapt. Transcend. Curious. Tolerant. Exist. Instinctual. Out of head. Into body.

I needed to immerse myself, conscience and confidence, into these themes if I wanted to achieve what *BFW—Birthing From Within—*calls the introspective "dream-like state of Laborland."

There was no *if* about it. Heck *yeah*, I wanted Laborland.

I had gone through neither a thirty-hour induced labor that resulted in a cesarean that further resulted in eight weeks of complications nor an eight-week long natural miscarriage to miss out on Laborland yet again.

If this child stays with us, if I carry to term, if I could successfully carry out an HBAC labor—like Clark W. Griswold's "Walley World"—if we got within "ten hours" of Laborland, then nobody is "bailing out. I'm gonna have fun and you're gonna have fun. We're all gonna have so much fucking fun..."

To get to Laborland, to realize my themes, just one theme held the key—surrender.

Yes, I can do that.

I winced tenderly with the thought, my palm splaying across an ever-growing abdomen, checking in with the thirteen-weeker I was carrying while commemorating the one we lost. The one who taught me surrender. The one who taught me that surrender is sometimes greater than resistance, notably in prevailing.

So strange, an oxymoron—surrender prevails.

*BFW* noted that "Women have to prepare for birth in their heart and soul, not their head."

I *was* preparing in my heart and soul, the Chant Sheet reverberating handpicked preparatory themes from my head to my heart, my soul, my body, my bones.

But...

Believing my body and my bones would and could do this was easier than getting downright frank about *how* my body and my bones were going to do so. *How* were they going to manage the pain?

I remember learning in nursing school that pain can be both objective and subjective. Objective pain symptoms, such as restlessness, pallor, rapid pulse, and rapid respiration, are perceptible not only to the individual feeling them but to others. However, the subjective aspect rules the pain roost, so to speak. If an individual says their pain is a 10—the worst possible pain—there is no objective measure that can prove otherwise. As emotional as it is sensory, and often very difficult to express in words, subjective pain depends a lot on the individual's physiological and psychological interpretation of pain.

Yes, in my first birth I found labor objectively the most rigorous type of physiological pain I had ever experienced. The psychological aspect of knowing that the contractions were going to come back again and again did not help matters. The hardest part was that it was seemingly unending, a marathon of pain.

Sure, I had been in pain before—a broken leg, a sprained ankle, delayed-onset muscle soreness from the occasional grueling workout. But none of them could hold a candle to labor. Even the two kidney stones I experienced in my early college years, surely from poor nutrition and poor hydration, with their lower back-burning, radiating knife-like nerve pain, and abrupt cold and clammy sweats with a side of vomitus, could not compete with labor. The quintessential example of subjective pain, some who withstood kidney stones would describe them as "pain worse than childbirth."

Yes, I objectively found labor to be unlike any other kind of pain. And I didn't even make it to the pushing phase in my first birth!

Labor *is* unlike any other kind of pain...in that the pain of labor is *not* in response to harm; nothing is wrong.

Passing a kidney stone through a ureter, through a urethra, in the end is not in the least bit rewarding—all of that pain for a pebble?

Passing a baby through a uterus, through a vagina, in the end is at least rewarding—all of that pain for a prize.

"Pain is purposeful," said *BFW*.

Pain in labor is part of "nature's blueprint" where "stretch receptors in the dilating cervix send signals to the brain, calling for more oxytocin to be released, which in turn fuels labor and increases dilation." Pain in labor is part of a positive feedback mechanism involving hormones and endorphins, both naturally pain-causing and pain-relieving. Pain in labor propels us toward instinct, toward the primitive brain, further propelling us into positions optimal for getting baby out. Understanding the basic concept that pain in labor is purposeful—full of intention—was the first step in my acceptance of that pain.

The pain *would* be there. I *would* have to find a way to cope with it.

Acknowledging that pain would be part of my labor and birth brought to mind another acknowledgment: pain had been part of labors and births for eons. It would hurt no more than I could stand. Other women, many with far less amenities than I enjoy in this century, had labored and birthed before me. They did it. They made it. They coped with the pain, laboring and birthing in unmedicated awareness.

Writer and filmmaker Suzanne Arms said of her childbirth activism "…the circumstances of our lives should be seen as valuable for helping us accomplish our life's purpose and bring forth our unique gifts. I think my gift had to do with my own wound, which was having such a traumatic birth." She also said, "Childbirth is an experience in a woman's life that holds the power to transform her forever. Passing through these powerful gates—in her own way—remembering all the generations of women who walk with her…She is never alone."

I *love* that. The generational thing. I wanted to be a part of that. That group of women. My grandmother, who gave birth to ten of her eleven children at home. It just screamed "bucket list" to me.

After grasping that pain in labor is not merely pain for the sake of pain but purposeful pain, I chose to willingly accept it as part of my birth experience. I could find common ground with the pain of childbirth; I could commit to being as determined as it was. The *why* of pain in birth savvied, I could move on to the *how*. How exactly was I going to cope with it? How would pain and I best work together to birth a child?

In my labor preparation, and specific to coping with pain in labor, I found invaluable *BFW*'s in-depth section on "Birthing Through Pain." In my paperback edition, sixty-five pages centered on the ecology of pain, beliefs and attitudes about pain, with at least twelve specific and proven pain-coping techniques, even an additive chapter on "the compassionate use of drugs and epidurals." I especially enjoyed the exercises and encouragement to try each of the pain-coping techniques, for the sake of finding which ones worked for me.

To this day I have not forgotten the techniques that I found advantageous—"Breath Awareness," "Finding Your Voice," and "The Communication of Touch."

Similar to chanting, I was familiar with "Breath Awareness" long before I realized I was familiar with breath awareness. As a vocalist and distance runner in high school, I can still recall the twenty-plus-years-gone-by guidance of my choir instructor and my track coach.

"Support your diaphragm, supporting your breath and pitch. Breathe deeply into your abdomen, filling it up and *out* as far as possible. On the exhale, the abdomen contracts in while the voice projects out. The diaphragm may be firm, but everything else...limbs, chest, shoulders, jaw...must stay relaxed."

"Breathe deeply. In through the nose and out the mouth. Use the abdomen—the diaphragm. Use your core to run. Shoulders, arms, hands relaxed. No clenching. Legs loose. Relax. Breathe. Run...through the pain. Find that runner's high."

Not only in singing and running but in laboring and birthing, something as simple and purposeful as breath is as essential in birthing life as it is essential to life. Relax. Breathe. Birth...through the pain. It is not easy, but with awareness it is doable and crucial, a distinct high.

"Finding Your Voice," with its chanting segue, surely appealed to me. More so than the chanting was the focus on a woman's "voice." Emphasis that all women have unique voices, such uniqueness further distinct in birth, a woman's "birthing voice" may surprise even herself. With the proposition that not all women respond to labor pain quietly, my attention was seized.

I distinctly remember while laboring with Mila that in the hospital room next door was a laboring woman who my mother may have deemed "a screamer." Although obvious, it didn't bother me much. Okay, maybe it scared me a smidge, wondering if that was soon to be my fate! What would hurt so bad that I would scream and keep on screaming?

And Mom had already mentioned in a previous conversation about labor how she did not understand what made some women "yell and scream and holler." "You're not going to be a screamer, are you?" she asked. Mom, who prefers to cope with pain discreetly, could not comprehend how that would help at all. In her opinion and experience, it would only make things worse by escalating the noise, the tension, the atmosphere.

No, I didn't want to be "a screamer"…did I?

"Finding Your Voice" disclosed for me an awareness of societal tendency—be it mine, my mother's, an institution's, the collective "our"—toward stoicism and encouraged me to reassess that. "…approach your birth with an openness to do whatever your body needs you to do. Don't make a prideful plan to labor quietly…vocalization through pain can be both a distraction and a release. When you hit your thumb with a hammer, you probably say 'Ouch!' or chant some profanity."

Yes! Yes! I do that!

You mean I can cuss in labor?

My affinity for "The Communication of Touch" pain-coping technique was quite surprising. Like many, I deal best with pain, physical and emotional, alone. And don't touch me, please. I don't want to cry or lash out. Now that's not stoic at all! Ay yi yi. But as *BFW* pointed out, "Some people want to be held and stroked during painful experiences, while others handle pain better when left alone. Regardless of your usual inclination, your needs in labor could be exactly opposite."

My needs in labor *were* exactly opposite. Regardless if he could do anything for me, Wade's presence in labor *was* reassuring. Whether massaging my lower back or holding my hand or propping me up while

I leaned on him or not touching me at all but simply being present, having him there *was* a comfort. No, I did not want to labor alone.

With some theoretical techniques under my belt, it was time to test the proof in the "pain cube."

The premise of *BFW*'s "Learning With Ice Cubes" exercise is to gauge "baseline response to pain" by using "pain cubes"—ice cubes—to simulate labor pain. Although the authors are candid about how *nothing* can truly simulate labor pain except labor pain.

So the exercise goes, you press an ice cube to a sensitive body part, such as the inner wrist or behind the ear, for sixty seconds to simulate a contraction. You can use one or two or more ice cubes—if you are a glutton for pain—and extend the length of the "contraction" to ninety seconds. While one's skin is exposed to the ice for the simulated contraction, she is encouraged to deploy her pain-coping techniques of choice.

First of all, "pain cube" is quite fitting. Holding the ice cube to my inner wrist for sixty seconds hurt a lot worse than I imagined it could. The pain felt to me like nerve pain—prickling, tingling, burning—very agitating, and in a way similar to the pain of labor and birth. Again, like many, I find nerve pain the most difficult to bear.

Secondly, my theoretical pain-coping techniques proved surprisingly effective. As I held the ice cube to my inner wrist, Wade deployed his "communication of touch" by massaging my lower back. Per *BFW*'s instruction, instead of focusing on the massage itself, I focused on my lower back and how good it felt in comparison to my inner wrist. I focused on redirecting my "breath awareness" to relax like my lower back rather than tense up like my inner wrist. I focused on "finding my voice," the innate groans and growls that released from my relaxed jaw released with themselves otherwise pent-up pain.

Sure, I could still feel the sting of the ice but it was muted, my mind preoccupied—distracted—with other things. The preparation, practice, repetition afforded efficacy in making it through frequent mock ice contractions.

Of course, Wade had to try the pain cubes...without a stitch of preparation. I told him, he should have read the book!

"Oh, babe, it's just ice. Give me one of those things." He pushes up the sleeve of his shirt, exposing a wrist nearly twice the girth of mine. A wrist that he fractured during a football game yet continued playing... all season long.

This isn't even going to touch him, I keep the deflating thought to myself as I direct him to the kitchen sink for pain cube runoff. Leveling your standard ice cube on his inner wrist, I deploy my version of intimidating football trash-talk, which comes in the form a Greek proverb: "It is drops of water that make a hole in the rock...hotshot." Then I promptly start the timer. Sixty seconds, a *nice* active contraction.

"Hmm, it's cold. Colder than I thought," he admits, looking over his shoulder at me...not even ten seconds in.

I stand behind him, arms crossed, leaning against the counter and raking the corner of my bottom lip through my teeth. I am conflicted. Is it natural to want your husband to writhe in pain? Come on, pain cube, I mutter internally, do your worst.

"Ba-a-abe..." his voice riddles with suspicion or maybe realization, "what'd you get me into?" He smiles the cutest little shit smile, an apology for the crow he is about to eat.

"It takes teamwork to make the dream work," I relish in saying back to him one of his signature quotes.

"Teamwork, my ass, this is a setup." He sways back and forth at the sink. "How long?"

"Twenty-two seconds."

"What?!"

I laugh—full-on cackle—unsure if it is more in amusement or satisfaction. "Here, let *me* rub *your* back," I wisecrack. But I do rub his back and coach a bit, "focus on your breathing."

"Aaarrrggghhh," he growls on a long exhale. "Damn, this stings." His brows arch, accentuated and convincing, as if he is telling me anything new! "How long?"

"Ten seconds longer than the last time you asked." My fingertips sink into the ticklish flesh of the V on his abdomen.

He laughs—not a full-on cackle but a foul-tasting chuckle, nonetheless—growling and swaying and squirming and hovering over the kitchen sink, demanding every ten seconds "How long?" until the last second passes. Until he can hurl the ice cube into the sink, taking great pleasure and great pains in crushing it up in the garbage disposal.

"Whoo! Babe. And you're gonna do that? Here? At home. No drugs."

"Yep," I do not hesitate, mind made up.

"You're the toughest woman I know." He pulls me into his chest for that hug only he can give.

Well, now don't I feel bad for wishing him writhing.

"How many of those, contractions, are you gonna have to go through?"

"A lot." I bury my head in his chest just thinking about it.

"One contraction every three to five minutes…twelve to twenty contractions per hour," he actually does the math.

I groan. Doesn't he know by now that math loathes me? And the feeling is mutual. "One!" I assert. "One contraction at a time. That's all we need to focus on."

"'Now o'clock,'" he agrees, proud of his recalling from my Chant Sheet.

We break our hold. I head for the bathroom to get brushed up for bed.

"So that was a contraction, huh," he calls after me.

"Ha!" I give him all the reply that question deserves.

"Okay, on a scale of one to ten, how do the ice cubes rate to a contraction?"

I shrug, having tried to accurately size up that question myself. Squeezing out a ribbon of toothpaste onto my toothbrush, I settle on, "Four? Maybe five."

"Five?" his tone deflates.

A fusion of *Tombstone* paraphrasing—one said to and one said by Val Kilmer's "Doc Holliday"—garbles over my toothpaste-laden tongue, "'My loving man, you're an oak.'"

"Uh-huh," he chuckles.

Standing behind me, his hands entwine themselves around the ever-expanding bump. He looks at our little triad in the mirror—bump, mama, daddy—eyes inevitably settling on the bump. There is that wonder again. I saw it in him during our pregnancy with Mila. It has returned. The same as attempting to conjure up some semblance of a contraction with the pain cube exercise, he wonders what it would be like to carry and grow and birth a child.

They'll just never know.

# The Lizard & The Lotus

NOT TO BE LEFT OUT, MILA PARTICIPATED IN THE *BIRTHING FROM WITHIN* activities, too.

"The Art of Birthing" section encourages exploration of the pregnant, laboring, and birthing self through art—painting, drawing, sculpting, even belly casting.

Stocked up on paint, brushes, and heavy-weight paper, we, my two-and-a-half year old and I, found refuge from the dog days of summer around a Minnie Mouse toddler table. The accompanying chairs' weight limit of seventy pounds, the bump and I felt like rebels!

With our ambient birthing playlist in chant mode too, providing a soundtrack, Mila and Mama painted until we ran out of expression…or until it was time to start dinner.

I am the first to admit that when it comes to drawing and painting, I have two left hands. Yes, I even gave the left hand a go, seeing how I find lefties especially artistic. Sad to say, it was equally as awkward.

Refusing to let that stop me, I painted and painted and painted, taking heed in *BFW*'s advice: "Some people think if they can't do something perfectly, they shouldn't do it at all. But in this exercise, as well as in your birth, it's your best effort that counts, not the attaining of some perfect image."

I gave it my best effort, and Wade could actually identify a few of the paintings.

"A lizard?" he half stated, half questioned.

"Yeah! You see that?" I half gloated.

It was supposed to represent my reptilian brain, the old and primitive and instinctive one. That shift from left brain to right brain, conscious to unconscious, the "birthing brain" would take me to Laborland.

If my primitive brain painting would resemble anything, I presumed it would resemble a cave painting—stick figure with a stick weapon, a warrior.

Eh, turns out I am more lizard than warrior.

In an attempt at being organic in the drawings, maybe I would give myself a subject or use one from *BFW*. Then I would just kind of zone out by rubbing the bump while watching Mila paint. My babies. What could be more inspiring? Mila's hands, still dimpled at the knuckles, I know them by heart. For not even one year later they will have evolved—more coordination, dexterity, mastering—until one day the dimpled knuckles will be no more.

Painting with her brought to my attention that I could stand to see things differently. With my approaching middle age, an A is an A, an n is an n, and an m is an m. In her toddlerhood, an A is a house, an n is a one-humped camel, and an m is a two-humped camel. And when she writes her letters and numbers, their origins may vary from traditional rules. Who says you have to write from left to right and top to bottom! When asked why she consistently drags out the "tail" of her lowercase α when spelling her name but not at any other time, she said, "Because I like it that way." Free of precedent, she is able to nurture the abstract.

Brush in hand, I followed her lead. Don't label. Don't preconceive. Don't draw the obvious.

It *was* offbeat, drawing lines and angles, wondering what—if anything—would form, only to end up with an amalgamation of triangles that appeared to be some sort of lizard-looking thing.

"Why the triangles?" I questioned, contemplating the lizard that was formed with them, after showing the painting to Wade.

"Strength," he said affirmatively, no half question this time.

"Huh?"

"They're sturdy, babe. You know, A-frame houses..." His arms made a triangle above his head, a rather large one considering his wingspan. My mind flickered to Mila and her houses made of A's; she has her daddy's eye. "...basic structure that bears a shit-ton of weight. Strength, babe, strength." He winked at me, believing in my strength more than I did.

I figured he should know, construction in his blood, but that didn't stop this old dog from digging.

As he said, triangles are iconic for their resistance to pressure—the strongest and most versatile geometric shape, the "geometry chameleon." Yep, a geometry lizard. Maybe math isn't so bad after all. I *would* need strength and pliability to birth this child.

The triangle effortlessly lends itself to the Trinity—Father, Son, and Holy Spirit—who I was convinced I would need even more than strength and pliability to pull off natural labor. And...in my research, I found that the triangle is an ancient symbol representative of the "genitalia of a goddess," representative of femininity—the "sacred triangle."

The oldest lizard is thought to be 240 million years old. I'd say that's ancient. Therefore, I saw no reason why ancient symbolism couldn't just as easily apply to the genitalia of a lizard.

"That looks like..." Wade tilted his head until it was nearly parallel to his shoulder before continuing, "a vagina inside a flower?"

"Yes!" I shouted, triumphantly.

"Open like a flower, birth from within," the paraphrase or quote—I lost track, taking so many notes—was on my Chant Sheet. And the Chant Sheet was within me, every drawing reflective of some grayscale-printed principle on standard white 8.5 X 11 background. If only I had known the Chant Sheet would be so incomparable, valuable, four pieces of flimsy paper I will keep forever, I would have created it with a bit more care.

It *was* a vagina inside a flower, a yellow lotus in bloom.

"In order to grow...first you must have the mud" is another paraphrased quote, as part of a larger whole, I scribbled onto yellow legal pad paper after reading that it inspired the title of Goldie Hawn's memoir *A Lotus Grows in the Mud*.

That was twelve years ago. I was living in Los Angeles. I was twenty-eight years old. Was I ever twenty-eight? I assumed the quote spoke to me, pertaining to personal music and acting endeavors. For the millions of us throwing hats into the music and acting arena in LA, there was plenty of mud!

Amazing is this circular universe.

My children were the furthest thing from my twenty-eight-year-old mind, convinced I likely wouldn't have any. My children are the most potent catalyst for personal growth I have ever experienced.

All of that soul-searching, years of it, when it would take something greater than myself—a focus other than myself, something worthy of growing up out of the mud for—to fully discover myself. Motherhood is proving to be my fast-track to self-discovery.

Each pregnancy, one birth and one miscarriage, has been uniquely different, revealing and cultivating in each its own right, but ultimately interconnected. Each, like the lotus, was symbolic of rebirth. Each, like the maturating lizard who loses her skin in patches or climbs out of it altogether and leaves it behind in one piece, was necessary for growth.

At the nucleus of my exploration, visualization, and preparation in my third pregnancy lies my ignorance about its importance in my first pregnancy, and the result thereof. Although, my second pregnancy ending in miscarriage, that provided the mud in which to grow. The first time I read *BFW*, days after a positive pee stick and days before a miscarriage, I skimmed over the entire art section. How is art going to help me labor and birth? That's kind of out there, even for me. Only after miscarrying, in all of that mud, did patience and humility then register. Pregnant for the third time, I read, slowly and determinedly, the art section two more times, genuinely participating, trying—growing.

And I must be way out there, because the art section became the most memorable section, as well as the most used. Dog-ears galore, the memories of a mother and a daughter spending together their last months of precious one-on-one time will forever bear-hug my heart.

A "Mila 2016" original is framed and hangs on our wall. The flood of sweet recollection it will bring in about twenty years, when my postmenopausal womb has long gone dormant, when Wade and I have pruned a bit more, when we are empty nesters. We will look at that vibrant painting, from the hand of a girl who will have bloomed—like the lotus and out of her own share of mud, and like the lizard with much skin sloughing and growth to experience—right under our noses into a full-grown woman and say, "Remember when…"

# You're Gonna What

WADE IS THE MOST PASSIONATE PROPONENT FOR HOME BIRTH.

He will share his enthusiasm with anyone who will listen. Therefore, on the off chance you run into my husband, do not bring up home birth unless you are in no particular hurry to get away from him.

Although...he was as skeptical as many at first.

"I just want you to be safe."

That is what most everyone said when I disclosed my intention for a home birth, an HBAC—home birth after cesarean—to be precise.

It is not as if I brought it up willingly for discussion. I purposely avoided putting it out there. I knew what the reaction would be.

People assume if you are pregnant, you are seeing a doctor and you are giving birth in a hospital. I get it. That is what we in the U.S., and growing numbers of other cultures, are accustomed to. And for those who desire it—and, of course, those who require it—I am deeply grateful that hospitals exist. It only would have been uplifting to feel as though others felt equally the same about my desire for a home birth.

Security: Some people build their lives around it. Some people build careers out of providing it. While others seek its antithesis, believing life begins outside the comfort zone.

While I gravitate toward the latter, believing the only walls that truly confine us are the ones we build around ourselves, no adrenaline junkie am I. A childhood spent riding the roller coaster of family dysfunction was all the *rush* I'll ever need. The only literal roller coasters I rode were Predator and Viper. I hated every millisecond of it. My eyes slammed shut, my hands clutching, my teeth gritting, the *young* ol' nag yelled the entire way. Why are we doing this! Because everyone else is! Stupid! Stupid! Stupid! I don't like this at all! You don't even like it! This is so not safe!

I didn't ride either roller coaster because I wanted to or because everyone else was. I rode the Predator to quell my curiosity. How else am I to know if it is all it's cracked up to be? I rode the Viper after finding out I detested the Predator, even more than I detested making my bed, because I said I would. Two, the Predator *and* the Viper, that was the deal...or double-dog dare, no doubt. On a school choir trip, I agreed to ride both roller coasters with my dearest and oldest friend. Oldest not eldest, she will appreciate and revel in my clarifying that. Crazy kid, she loved roller coasters so much, she rode them both again and again.

And there you have it...aside from one's physical security...safety is subjective. What two people consider safe can be as divergent as their taste in music.

Take for instance my four station safety barometer: Hell No, Heck Yeah, Maybe, Never Again.

Climbing Mount Everest—Hell No. #brrrhhh!

Skydiving—Heck Yeah.

*Running Wild with Bear Grylls*—Maybe.

Roller coaster—Never Again.

The bucket list barometer could go on and on. The same as yours could. And how different would they be? How different would risk assessment be?

"I never could have done that. You're braver than I!" said many a hospital-birther to a homebirther.

To which the homebirther retorted, "Oh, no, you're the brave one!"

Somewhere in the semantics, both women wonder, what did she mean by "brave"?

Brave...as in courageous?

Or...brave...as in dumb.

Or...worse yet...brave...as in irresponsible...as in reckless...as in endangering the life of an unborn child.

Whether rational or polarizing, the greater point in the birth safety debate is that there is no such thing as "safe" or "risk-free" birth in any setting.

It is no less brave than it is reckless to birth a child in a hospital.

It is no less brave than it is reckless to birth a child at home.

It *is* a choice.

A choice that deserves as much encouragement as any other choice, a choice that seems to me not merely overlooked but excluded, not even considered.

Growing up in rural Pennsylvania, the Amish horse-drawn buggy could potentially be a daily sighting. I didn't know much about the Amish. I knew they made killer banana nut bread. I knew they dressed funny. Yes, I can say that because they thought I dressed funny, too, as evidenced by a group of Amish girls tee-hee'g and pointing at my stone-washed denim skirt, neon pink tank top, and jelly shoes at the local quick mart whilst they were covered from neck to toe in billowy black garb in the heat of summer and mounting up in a horse-drawn buggy. My '80s teenage attitude begged, who should be laughing at whom! And I knew they delivered their babies at home. A neighbor told me they used his phone to call for "help." I did not know, however, that help was a midwife. All I knew was, who has babies at home? As if!

Overlooked. Excluded. Not even considered.

Then, twenty-some years later and inspired to consider home birth, it seemed others were considering me, and my choice, at best "different" and at worst "unsafe."

Could I blame them? Not even a decade ago, fresh out of nursing school, if you would have told me that I would give birth at home, I would have cackled you out of the hospital I was working in!

Overlooked. Excluded. Not even considered.

What makes one choice different where another choice, still just a choice at its root, is what? Common, standard, normal, better, safer? When the one making a different choice likely considers it the best choice, maybe even an extension of who they are. Like Nelson Mandela said, "May your choices reflect your hopes, not your fears."

Home birth *is not* different; it *is* a choice.

It seems peculiar to me that many are still debating the safety of home birth, when legend has it there are cultures who used to birth babies in the sea and some still birth babies in special rivers and natural shallow waters.

I cannot be the only one who gets a thrill out of imagining where babies were born throughout history—Stonehenge before it was "Stonehenge," Yellowstone before it was "Yellowstone," the Amazon, the Sahara, the Andes—when home was where the uterus was, so to speak.

But oftentimes I felt like the only one.

It was hard not to feel that way when most in my circle responded with knee-jerk objection: "You're gonna what?"

Of course, their concern stemmed from love. I understood that. And, in their hearts, they all wanted for me the birth experience that I desired.

I just never heard anything remotely close to "I've heard wonderful things about home birth. What a fantastic decision. How important it is to have that choice. How sweet it is that Mila will be a part of it." It was more of a "fingers crossed, I hope you get what you want and that everybody is safe" support. And, ultimately that was enough. I was thankful for any support, regardless of its motivation. I simply could not recall that sense of concern suppressing excitement with our hospital birth.

Regardless of what I wanted, the people who loved me wanted for me a safe birth. Whether via experience and/or convention, it was a simple formula: hospital birth = safe, home birth = *What* is home birth?

So I let those that love me undertake the fearing and the worrying. I should have thanked them, because they did enough of it that I didn't have to.

The ol' nag brayed. The bottom line is…it's my body, my baby, my birth…butt out! But I listened, to the worries, the counterarguments, the questions, consciously attempting to hear their opinions, acknowledge their feelings, and share my own recently acquired.

It only further cemented my dedication, having people question me. And, in the meantime, if I propelled anyone to examine their view of birth and how and where it is to be done, well, then, chalk one up for me.

I wished I had more to give them. I wished I had some generational, communal "women who have done it supporting and guiding others through it" fairy tale to tell:

My mother, the last of eleven and the first to be born in a hospital, would have been born at home, too. Mom would have birthed me and my sisters at home. Generation after generation, clinging boldly to privilege and amenity, the women in our family and circle of friends would have birthed in the intimacy of homes, allowed to witness the power and transformation of birth without medical distraction. Generation after generation, we would have an inherent and inherited learning of labor and birth. We would understand the significance of that rite and that right. When it came time for my first birth with Mila, I would have known what to do, *what to expect...*

# Data...Yawn

IN THIS INFORMATION AGE, ANYONE CAN FIND ANYTHING THAT SUPPORTS THEIR sensibilities. If June believes hospital birth is safer than home birth, there are studies and reports and information abound to support June's belief. If January believes home birth is safer than hospital birth, there are studies and reports and information abound to support January's belief. Naturally, September believes the truth lies somewhere in the middle.

What are we to believe, exactly?

Science that supports our theories? Potentially skewed science that supports our theories?

Why are many in the medical community quick to debunk anecdotal evidence—evidence collected in a casual or informal manner and relying heavily or entirely on personal testimony; based on personal experience—when the scientific method, with all its empirical and measurable data, can yield varying outcomes/statistics dependent upon who is doing the study, who is paying for the study, and what point is up for proving?

When you are in search of a new book to read, a new show to binge watch, a fine dining experience, which carries more weight—systematic reviews or word of mouth?

Novelist and poet Gertrude Stein was ahead of her time when in 1946 in reference to why she "had not been able to take any interest" in the Atomic Bomb said, "Everybody gets so much information all day long that they lose their common sense. They listen so much that they forget to be natural."

Wherefore...

In pursuit of a VBAC, I attempted to take it all in—evidential, scientific, anecdotal, medical, anthropological, quantitative, qualitative, et cetera—while hoping common sense would help me sort through it, resulting in a natural decision for me.

Certainly my first labor and birth got in the way of complete objectivity. How could it not?

Regardless, I learned a bit about myself, beyond birth preferences even. Although I have a medical background, I am more inclined to the anthropological than the medical. Anthropology speaks to something in me. I do not know exactly why, yet I know that I desire to be a part of that thread of existence, where even in a modern age I can strive to do certain things in a manner of my ancestors. Even if it is harder, longer, out of fashion.

Although a central lesson in my Master's education was that the scientific method is crucial in observing, analyzing, and concluding, the anecdotal has a greater overall impact on me and my perspective. Birth stories affected me, stayed with me, far beyond any scientific study I read.

In that Master's schooling, qualitative research inspired me, where I was convinced quantitative research with all its measurable, mathematical, statistical data…yawn…was only always one study shy of boring me to tears. Be that as it may, quantitative research is what drove the point home in regard to hospital birth, supporting the safety and efficacy of home birth, HBAC precisely.

When comparing stats, no significant difference was found in adverse neonatal outcomes between hospital birth and planned home birth, particularly when integrative systems of care and support were in place, such as hospital transport if necessary. Adverse maternal outcomes and rates of birth intervention were significantly lower in planned home birth populations. Merely one of many examples, the national cesarean rate of thirty-plus percent for women birthing in hospitals decreases to five percent for women birthing at home with a midwife. In regard to TOLAC—trial of labor after cesarean—studies show midwifery-led HBACs have the highest success rate (87%).[1] And in-hospital midwifery-led VBACs achieve higher success rates (61.2%) than those led by obstetricians (46.9%).[2]

Of course, one could argue the fact that midwives do not see the high-risk patients that obstetricians do. I could pose the inverse. Being a low-risk patient with both pregnancies, how is it I birthed naturally at home with a midwife but ended up with nearly every intervention on the menu, ultimately a cesarean, in the hospital with an obstetrician?

I personally found it is sensible to consider the quantitative cost-benefit analysis, not simply to the woman and her family but to society at large. Convincing every pregnant woman she needs to birth in a hospital may be lucrative for the medical, pharmaceutical, and insurance industries. My hospital birth—where my choices did not lead my birth experience—was billed at thirty-plus thousand dollars. My home birth—where my choices did lead my birth experience—was billed at three-plus thousand dollars. Taking into account deductibles, what was actually paid out followed suit with insurance covering thirteen thousand for our hospital birth and thirteen hundred for our home birth. If you have already done the math, that is a nine hundred percent difference. *Nine hundred percent.*

It seemed to me as much a responsible, sound, important thing to do as recycling. Yes, if I—low-risk mama—wanted to and could, I should.

Call me January, but I found the quantitative further backed by the qualitative in birth stories comparing hospital and home birth. Hands down, efficacy—producing the labor and-birth experience desired by the laboring and birthing woman—seemed to be on the side of the homebirther.

# Nurses On Horseback

HOME BIRTH WAS THE ARCHETYPE; WOMEN WERE THE ARCHITECTS.

For eons, women inherited birth knowledge from each other, handing down experience from mother to daughter and from neighbor to neighbor. "Wise women," as those with certain learning and skills were often called by the community, were the first caregivers, providers, obstetricians, one could say, to pregnant and birthing women and their newborns.

Long before its association with being married, the term "wife" meant "woman." Add "mid"—"together with"—and you get "midwife," plainly translating to "with woman." As far back as ancient Egypt, midwifery was recognized as a "unique, social and female vocation...an artistic and autonomous profession supported by advanced and scientific knowledge."[1]

Some 5,000 years later and after the war of 1812, under the weight of social influence and frank sexism, midwives' intelligence and capability came into question with physicians, and other authorities, postulating concern that midwifery perpetuated "uneducated" and "indecent" ways.[2]

By the turn of the century, and in large part due to the organization and influence of the birth dictators, an institution, a holistic and cultural and evolutionary art—midwifery—had taken a hit.

By 1900, physicians were attending 50% of births in this country to include nearly 100% of births to middle-class and upper-class women. Yet less than 5% of women were birthing in hospitals with 95% still birthing at home. I guess, then, it is safe to surmise that even for obstetricians home birth was the archetype.

Those who promoted the idea that midwives were uneducated need look no further than the 1910 Flexner Report—however controversial and consequential it is now viewed in modern times—which revealed that 90% of doctors did not have college educations and that the 10% who did attended substandard medical schools. The report singled out obstetrics, noting, "But the very worst showing is made in the matter of obstetrics." Albeit backhandedly, it further elaborated, "...the student gets about the same training as a midwife."[3]

By 1920, over 30% of women gave birth in hospitals.

It was in this year that Dr. Joseph DeLee, who would become known as "the father of modern obstetrics," published an article that states, "It always strikes physicians as well as laymen as bizarre, to call labor an abnormal function, a disease, and yet it is a decidedly pathologic process." Sedation, episiotomy, forceps, placenta extraction, and induction became standard as DeLee was not the only obstetrician who believed "normal" deliveries to be rare. Yet, oddly enough, DeLee promoted the home birth setting as safe, cost effective, and practical—a beneficial training model for student doctors and nurses in "noninterventionist practices." In what DeLee considered an "outpatient" service, exceptional results were achieved with modest resources. His home-based/noninterventionist training model produced maternal and infant mortality rates consistently lower than those of the nation.[4]

By the late 1930s, 50% of all women and 75% of urban women birthed in hospitals. In the 1930s and in hospitals throughout the country, "twilight sleep"—which replaced chloroform as an anesthetic in childbirth—was standard protocol. In hindsight, some consider twilight sleep as violence against women, the injection inducing a state of disorientation that managed pain via amnesia rather than providing true analgesic pain relief. Women were often shackled, tied down, and padded because of violent hallucinations where they might thrash and bang wildly—arms, hands, feet, legs, head, anything loose enough to flounder—driven into a frenzy by the narcotics in their system and the pain, which they were very much experiencing but would not remember.

Paraphrasing a birth story from this era, the birthing mother recalled, "When I woke, they said, 'Here's your baby.' And I said, 'Oh, it is?'" No control. No participation. No recollection of birthing one's child? Not to mention the depressive central nervous system effects twilight sleep had on newborns that could result in drowsiness and respiratory distress.

A more humanistic way existed, even in 1925, as exhibited by Mary Breckinridge who founded the Frontier Nursing Service in Hyden, Kentucky, serving neglected women and children in the rural region of the Appalachian Mountains. Breckinridge, a graduate of St. Luke's Hospital Training School for Nurses in New York, joined the American Committee for Devastated France, working with midwives in providing help and medical care to those starving in French villages in the aftermath of World War I. It was this experience that propelled Breckinridge to view midwifery services as a "logical solution to many health problems in her own country." Completing midwifery training in Woolwich, England, Breckinridge returned to Kentucky where she helped establish the Kentucky Committee for Mothers and Babies. Later renamed the FNS, it was the first organization in the U.S. to use midwives under the direction of a single medical doctor, a collaborative and effective system that is still in use today.[5]

Those midwives, often called "nurses on horseback," traversed the remote mountainous Appalachian area by horseback. The image of midwives saddling through mountains became the subject of lore: When mountain children asked where babies came from, they were told, "The nurses bring them in their saddlebags." Nurses on horseback spent as much time traveling to and from patients' homes as they did in patients' homes, which is saying a lot because once labor started those midwives did not leave the patient, staying day in and day out if needed, until the child was born. And they did it all—prenatal care, birth, and ten days of postpartum care—for five dollars.

For one dollar more per family per year, general medical care and vaccinations could be provided by those midwives turned "family nurse," the sole family medical provider.

By 1932, it was reviewed and concluded by Metropolitan Life Insurance Company that "…the type of service rendered by the Frontier Nurses safeguards the life of mother and babe. If such a service were available to the women of the country generally, there would be a saving of 10,000 mothers' lives a year…30,000 less stillbirths and 30,000 more children alive at the end of the first month of life."[6]

There were obstetricians who advocated uninterrupted birth practices, too. The 1940s would see the groundbreaking publication of Dr. Grantly Dick-Read's book *Childbirth Without Fear: The Principles and Practice of Natural Childbirth*. The 1950s and 1960s would see the popularization of the Lamaze method and the Bradley method. The development of Dr. Fernand Lamaze's psychoprophylactic method was inspired by natural childbirth practices in the Soviet Union, which involved breathing and relaxation techniques under the supervision of a "monitrice"—a trained woman, similar to a midwife and/or a doula. Dr. Robert A. Bradley's method encouraged birthing women to trust their bodies, to "do the things that animal mothers do instinctively," and pioneered the inclusion of birth partners in the birthing process.

Midwives clung to their, and birthing women's, rights. By the 1950s, the midwifery division of the National Organization for Public Health Nursing developed its own philosophy that emphasized pregnancy and childbirth as a "normal process," as well as a family-centric event. The American College of Nurse Midwives was formed. Sloane Hospital for Women in New York City became the first mainstream medical institution to open its doors to nurse-midwives. By the 1970s, the U.S. military began training and using nurse-midwives.

Society kept pace. The civil rights movement, second wave of women's rights, Patient's Bill of Rights, consumer movement, and back-to-nature and health-food movement all had some momentum/criticism—a call for change—over medical management of childbirth throughout the 1960s and 1970s. It would be these grassroots efforts that would push for the "demedicalization" of childbirth, the legalization of midwifery and home birth, and the compromise between home and hospital birth with the rise of freestanding "birth centers."

Although, there was much recouping of rights and much work yet to be done. By 1960, 97% of births occurred in hospitals.

Ina May Gaskin, "the mother of modern midwifery," offered more than just natural birth at The Farm, which was more than just a farm, more than just a birthing center. Settled in rural Tennessee in

1971, The Farm was a community, an experience, a way of life. The Farm Midwives attended nearly 3,000 naturally laboring and birthing women—to include breech, twin, and VBAC births—with favorable statistics unseen by those in medical obstetrics at the time, and remain unseen by those of modern medical obstetrics. Spanning thirty years, The Farm's cesarean rate was less than 2%, their intervention rate via vacuum extraction and/or forceps delivery was less than 0.5%, their maternal mortality rate was 0%, and their intact perineum rate was an astounding 68.7%.[7] We are commonly told to expect the inverse, where the American College of Obstetricians and Gynecologists estimates that 53% to 79% of vaginal deliveries will result in laceration.

The 1980s did not see any surplus in home or birthing center births with out-of-hospital births representing just 1% in the "decade of excess." All the while a growing sense of crisis regarding adequate and effective maternity and reproductive health care for women plagued the country. Minority women, rural women, and women facing socio-economic disadvantage were affected the most, routinely lacking access to adequate care. Midwives, often under threat of persecution and/or prosecution, had served those very women not even a half century ago. Midwives could have been part of a solution had they not been restrained by red tape.

Progressively and on the bright side, midwives are becoming a legitimate part of the solution. It seems peculiar even putting it that way, considering that for the largest share of our history babies were born into the hands of midwives. Only over the course of the past few centuries has it become commonplace for them to be born into the hands of obstetricians.

The American College of Obstetricians and Gynecologists projects an ob-gyn shortage of 8,000 by 2020 and 22,000 by 2050. The shortage multifaceted, there is obviously a shortage of midwives, too; there has been for some time, no thanks to the powers that be. With just over 11,000 midwives and 20,000 ob-gyns, half of the counties in the U.S. are still in need of a midwife, an ob-gyn, a single reproductive care provider.[8]

Other countries, and even forward-thinking hospitals in this country, have found that by utilizing midwives alongside obstetricians, they can better serve pregnant and birthing women, even better serve women's health in general. An efficacious model that results in increased patient education, choice, and satisfaction while decreasing intervention and cost is a basic collaborative effort where high-risk women see obstetricians and low-risk women have the option of seeing midwives.

As more women become informed of and empowered by their prenatal and birthing options, and as more legislation, states, and insurance providers fully support those options, the demand and availability of midwives is rising. According to the National Center for Health Statistics, the percentage of midwife-attended births in the U.S. has risen nearly every year since 1989, or at least remained steady. From 2004 to 2012, in certain states midwifery saw a 50% increase in out-of-hospital births.[9] In 2014, midwives attended 8% of all births—some out of hospital, more in hospital. The Bureau of Labor Statistics reports the number of nurse-midwives has increased by 30% since 2012.

Maybe the pendulum swings back.

Another historical irony?

Midwives, once nearly driven into obscurity by the demands of the birth dictators, may very well be the key to meeting the demands of a well-known shortage in reproductive care providers.

Similar to those mysterious nurses on horseback, in modern times one could think of midwifery as a dark horse—a little known contender that makes an unexpectedly good showing.

# Nesting

If ever I nested with baby girl, it must have been subliminal.

Maybe it was due to the disconnect between home preparation and hospital birth. With the exception of having everything ready for baby to come home, and without planning on laboring and birthing at home, there was not much to plan.

Somewhere in that disconnect was the certainty that I was oblivious to the importance of birth preparation. There *was* much to plan. Wade and I were equally clueless about how having a child was going to change our life. A new mother and a new father, attempting to maintain habits and freedoms of the old life with the new life, were surprised and a bit disenchanted when the two did not flawlessly mesh. Sooner or later, we realized our firstborn was the new life—the new lifestyle—being bound to her sweeter than any freedom we ever tasted.

Child and family centric by the time my belly flourished with baby boy, I could feel myself hunkering down early in the second trimester.

*This* is nesting!

I found nesting to have much in common with a "five senses" activity.

In one fell swoop, I completed homework from Genevieve that turned into "sight nesting" by envisioning birth in every possible way in our home. Every room, every position, in the water, out of the water, in the bed, on the floor, no birth unseen. I even envisioned a hospital transfer…just once…in case that is what it came down to.

Literal and a bit figurative "sight-touch nesting," I plastered our walls with evocative pictures—mostly wall art collages illustrating Mila's striking growth from a seed in my womb to a sapling, and a few of Wade and I on our honeymoon, the beginning of our family. Anything left uncovered became wall art Chant Sheets, basically, which for my personal soul cup consisted mainly of scripture:

"I am the daughter of a king who is not moved by the world for my God is with me and goes before me; I do not <u>fear</u> because I am his." "She is clothed in strength and dignity, and she laughs without <u>fear</u> of the future." "Be strong and courageous. Do not be <u>afraid</u>; do not be discouraged, for the Lord your God will be with you wherever you go."

I wanted to come to grips with the theme of my hospital birth—what if, fear. I wanted to see the word "fear" staring back at me for twenty-six weeks. When it came time to birth, I wanted to be so accustomed to fear that I did not fear it. When—if—it showed up in my home birth, I would not give in to it. I would not operate out of it. I would stay the course, believing in myself and my body.

"Sound nesting" at its core, a portable speaker filled with ten hours plus of a laboring and birthing looping playlist was most touching to this nester. Believing in and having experienced music's capacity to make more tolerable inconvenient aspects of a task, I knew it would only enhance my physical and mental endurance in labor.

Unlike my first birthing playlist, I actually deliberated over this one. Neither workout songs nor cheeky songs such as *Push It* made the cut. Labor was not a party. I knew that now. Labor is its very definition: work, make great effort. Birth is an experience, a journey, a revolutionary road trip without wheels. Regardless of how I would arrive, the passage would not be wasted this time. The music would, and still does, provide a spellbinding score. Ever swelling and withdrawing, like the curves and slopes of a road, like the contractions of birth, the playlist kindled in me tenacity and tenderness, peace and power.

Many of the songs I turned to during my miscarriage made their way onto that playlist. Ray LaMontagne, Bob Dylan, Native American drum and chant, New Age meditation and nature sounds, I carry them in my solar plexus—the pit of my stomach—the way I still carry the one that got away.

Have you ever heard a mom say she feels like her children are still a part of her even though she gave birth years ago? Well, that's because it's true. With the advancement of DNA testing, scientists have concluded fetal cells can cross the placenta and enter mom's body, becoming part of her tissues. A phenomenon widespread among mammals, we mothers carry unique genetic material from each of our children's bodies within our body, creating what biologists call a "microchimera—named after the legendary beasts made of different animals."[1] Of course, scientists are excited about this premise, as they want to explore how those unique genetic materials affect the mother's tissues and health. I merely like the thought of my babies eternally living within me, if only their DNA.

What I consider sensual songs that I never thought to include in my first birthing playlist were intrinsic this go-round. Ed Sheeran's *Thinking Out Loud*, Sean Hayes' *Powerful Stuff*, and Eric Church's *Like a Wrecking Ball*—not to be confused with naked Miley riding one—easily made the cut. Even some old schoolers like Percy Sledge, Otis Redding, and Taj Mahal—not to be confused with the "wonder," although he is one— were shoo-ins.

The sensuality aspect came in reading birth stories that introduced to me the notion of the pleasure of childbirth, where couples kissed and caressed their way through contractions and/or birth. The documentary *Orgasmic Birth: The Best-Kept Secret* captures the essence that "labor and birth can be pleasurable—even ecstatic." In watching the film, I interpreted "orgasmic" in the figurative sense of an empowering and satisfying birth experience. However, I do not doubt that women are capable of literal orgasm in childbirth as I read in a few birth stories. As Ina May Gaskin plainly said, "The energy that gets the baby in is the energy that gets the baby out."

Whilst I was not able to capitalize on the literal orgasm for the literal pain, there *was* an ecstasy about delivering my child's body. That final push, knowing the pain was behind us and he was here with us on the outside, that we had made it, was nothing if not rapturous.

Those sensual songs served as a key reminder during hard labor that it is worth it, that I would do it all again, for Wade, for our child—a child made in and born out of love, passion, want, desire.

I included some Eagles, some Lionel Richie, and a little Willie, of course. We *were* birthing a Texan. Whitney's *My Love Is Your Love*, Alicia's *No One*, some gospel, pretty much the entire *P.S. I Love You* soundtrack, *Somewhere Over the Rainbow*, *What a Wonderful World*, anything I categorize as "easy listening" was fair game.

It wouldn't have been complete without some full circle listens. Chris Stapleton's *Traveller*, CCRs *Long as I Can See the Light*, and Pat Green's *Wave on Wave*—a little ditty I like to call *Wade on Wave*, so cheesy, I know—reminded me of how I got here, from "me" to "we."

Mila rounded out the playlist with her faves, only fitting as she would be a part of the birth. Jake Reese's *Day To Feel Alive* proved a nice uplifting addition. "I find my soul re*bible*"—aka revival—she sang to Maren Morris' *My Church*. And my fave of her faves was hearing her soft soprano voice match that of the chanting/singing children "Sa Ta Na Ma, I am the light of my soul..." from the *Children Beyond* soundtrack featuring Tina Turner.

If cows actually come home after an indefinite long time, they would be in our backyard as much as we have listened to that playlist. It, like the Chant Sheet, is a keepsake forever linking us to the nostalgia of planning and carrying out the birth of our son in our home and in our bed. It is dangerous, more like tempting, the feeling it evokes. Playlist crooning while preparing a special end-of-workweek feast, nip of wine easily heightening the sentimentality of it all, Wade nuzzles my neck, "Dontcha wanna have another one?" To which my chuckle matches his tone, somewhere between half joking and half considering.

Moving on to bona fide "touch nesting," I found my daily dose of TLC in a birthing hammock. Having played around with yoga hammocks for strength training and flexibility, I knew they provided a weightlessness similar to water yet uniquely different. Installing one at home was nothing a little rappelling equipment couldn't do. From a heavy duty ceiling hook that Wade shored up with a joist in the attic, I hung a 5/16" carabiner with a working load limit of 500 pounds, followed by a safety rotational device with a working load limit of 1,000 pounds, then one more carabiner, and at last a figure 8 descender, through which I rigged a sky blue 5.5 x 3 yard silk hammock with a 2,000 pound weight capacity.

Ahhh…heaven, pure antigravity-lower-back-loves-you-sky-blue-hammock relief!

If you Google "birthing hammock," you won't find much. Or maybe you will, requiring little to be a better Googler than I. The idea came to me, naturally, from *Birthing From Within*. I kept turning back to the page of a drawing of a woman squatting and birthing over a hammock. A primitive hammock, low to the ground and held up at both ends between stacks of heavy rocks, the child is born into the soft cloth. Mayan communities have used such hammocks "to aid mothers throughout pregnancy and childbirth for centuries."

I neither imagined that type of hammock nor birthing into one. What I could see was an aerial-like hammock, myself wrapped and supported in it, laboring and squatting, elongating the torso and keeping it upright to make good use of gravity. Arms and shoulders looped within, and upper back supported, the hammock could be used to take a burden off the legs in resting squat position below. Even looped underneath the breasts and above the bump, body in hands and knees position, the hammock could help relieve the burden of weight on the limbs. I used it this way in early labor, and I used it even more in the weeks and months before labor began.

My nightly ritual was to come straight from the bath into the hammock. Oh, I have waited for you all day! If you have never used a yoga or aerial hammock, please do not mistake it for a hammock that you hang between two trees. It is not that. It is larger and pliable—sweeping and draping from the ceiling. The closest thing to a second skin I have ever experienced, and much like a womb to a babe, it is cocooning. It is silky and smooth and rich and cool…the center of crème brûlée.

I rotated inside that hammock like a marshmallow on a stick at a beach bonfire, *roasting* the longest on my belly. While I am not a frequent stomach sleeper, in pregnancy I forgot how nice it was to at least have the option. That hour of nightly hammock heaven was pure bliss. Gently swaying back and forth—intermittently around in circles at

Mila's piloting—my lower back, and bones in general, were grateful for the reprieve. I have to think that it only helped in persuading baby into preferred anterior position as well. If my stomach was the "hammock" and my back was the "tree," what better way to encourage baby's back and bottom into the hammock than by lying on my stomach in a hammock, which allowed me to do so carefully by evenly distributing my weight and avoiding direct pressure on my abdomen.

Engulfed in sky blue, I relaxed. I visualized. It was surreal at times lying in that hammock with a child in my womb when I would think about my own childhood where I used to lay staring up at a sky of blue, mesmerized by the calm, the trust, the freedom it represented. So I envisioned delivering our child with that same sense of calm, trust, freedom. I envisioned delivering our child into it with the hope that he or she would not have to look so far to find calm, trust, freedom…the way mama did.

When the female bird nests, she gathers twigs, leaves, moss, grass, even *herbs* and spices. I, too, gathered—birthing props, massage cream, essential oils, a thirty-two hour apothecary candle with the hope of birthing long before it went out, even *herbs*, although no spices.

Fleshing out the senses project was "taste and smell nesting." Per Genevieve's recommendation, and having a mind to after a bit of research, I turned to specific and small quantity loose-leaf herbs ingested in tea form—"herbal infusions"—said to support prenatal health and wellness. Not only do specific herbs provide supplemental vitamins and minerals beneficial to the prenatal period, some actually provide medicinal actions beneficial to the prenatal period.

For instance, safely used as a "uterine tonic and general pregnancy tea" for at least two centuries—"wise women" may argue for thousands of years—red raspberry leaf has been shown to increase blood flow to the uterus and strengthen uterine muscle fibers, which promotes organized/effective contractions during labor, further improving labor outcome by reducing the need for medical intervention and preventing excessive bleeding after birth.[2]

When the postal service delivered our home birth kit, the first thing I searched for and pulled from the box was a tin canister of Happy Mama Herbals postpartum sitz bath.[3] A mixture of uva ursi, comfrey leaf, yarrow, sage, and calendula blossoms, my postpartum perineum would thank the wise women responsible for handing down the age-old remedy. Not only medicinal, indeed it was soothing, too. Those mama birds gathering herbs to build nests do so to help fight off bacteria, in a way scientists have yet to completely understand.[4]

Isn't it interesting how "natural" often gets thrown around in its relation not only to birth but to many things. It almost loses its significance, when "natural" is what ties us to nature, that which essentially relates us all—humans *and* birds nesting.

Another souvenir, there are moments when I cannot resist popping the top off of that tin canister. It takes only one deep inhale to transport me back in time, the redolent scent of the earthy herbs forever reminding me of a jubilant home birth.

Gratitude manifests in my smiling eyes, gratitude to a midwife and her apprentice who steeped those herbs then ladled them into home-made herbal ice packs and peri bottles. It is a gracious thing, to schlep oneself and supplies into another's home, taking care of and making convenient for another her labor and birth and postpartum healing. That kindness tucked away in a tin canister, ever so often released, wafts through my olfactory like chicken soup for the soul, releasing with it a surge of warmth and love to a midwife and her apprentice who took care of me at quite possibly the most vulnerable moments of my life.

The nesting/bird/herb/nature theme is significant of a conglomerate of quotes by arguably the most famous midwife Ina May Gaskin:

"Human female bodies have the same potential to give birth as well as aardvarks, lions, rhinoceri, elephants, moose, and water buffalo. We are the only species of mammal that doubts our ability to give birth. It's profitable to scare women about birth. But let's stop it. I tell women: Your body is not a lemon. Even if it has not been your habit throughout your life so far, I recommend that you learn to think positively about your body. (We are)...no more unsuited to give birth than any other of the 5,000 or so species of mammals on the planet. We are merely the most confused."

Another fusion of Ina May's quotes brings us full circle on Part II: *the learning*, which for me felt like *doing* nothing but was everything… essential:

"When you destroy midwives, you also destroy a body of knowledge that is shared by women, that can't be put together by a bunch of surgeons or a bunch of male obstetricians, because physiologically, birth doesn't happen the same way around surgeons (male or female), medically trained doctors, as it does around sympathetic women. Simply put, when there is no home birth in a society, or when home birth is driven completely underground, essential knowledge of women's capacities in birth is lost to the people of that society—to professional caregivers, as well as to the women of childbearing age themselves."

Nesting complete, and with the attending of a midwife who was not confused but very clear on women's capacities in birth, I was about to capture some of that essential knowledge.

# III

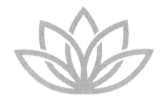

*the realizing*
*doing nothing is*
*doing everything*

# I Know A Little Something

They're coming. Contractions. And I know what to do.

*Do* nothing.

At this point, I would consider myself a well-read pregnant woman. *They* were right: some of it did scare me. But more than that, it conditioned me, readied me in mind and body, and whipped me into shape, so to speak.

This is not expecting. This is not pregnancy. This is labor. This is birth. I am prepared for this.

Surrender. Trust. Accept.

I rake the corner of my bottom lip through my teeth. Those teeth want to celebrate with a megawatt smile. They want to aid my tongue in shouting, We made it, baby! You stuck! But they are a tad preoccupied. Keeper of the floodgates, they instead aid my quivering lip that holds back tears of remembrance and appreciation and realization.

Fear and expectation—the themes of my first birth—have no place here. I embark on this birth with nothing but curiosity and awe.

Will we labor all day? Two days? More? Less? Will we welcome a girl? A boy? Will I crawl around on the floor? Will I curse? Will I scream? Will we birth in the tub? Squatting from the birthing hammock? On the floor? In the bed?

"Will" not "how."

Sure, both terms pose questions. But they do so with entirely different motivation and intention.

I am in *my* bed, our bed, where we conceived this child that is starting to knock ever so lightly on birth's door. Nothing about this bed feels remotely mechanical. I am warm of body and heart in *my* pajamas and beneath our sheets. Gown and sheets neither feel nor appear clinical in any way. There is no disruption, no rush, because there is nowhere to rush. No hospital bag to pack. No cold to schlep ourselves or a hospital bag out into. No red-eye drive. No rushing Mila off or calling someone in for a sleepover, only to return days later with a newborn in arms and no experience for her to grasp where the new baby came from.

Mila is in her bed, next to ours. She is warm, in her pajamas and beneath her sheets. She sleeps, uninterrupted, hopefully having the sweetest of dreams. Baby has a surprise for her. Wrapped and stowed away months ago to be given to "Big Sis" promptly after baby enters her world is a "Big Buck."

A close second to *Spirit*, Big Sis adores the animated film *Home on the Range*, featuring "Buck" the horse. Ergo, in her world, every horse is a "buck." Good luck explaining to her that a male deer is in fact a buck!

Baby is bringing Big Buck, a rather large stuffed horse. Big Sis immediately fell in love with Big Buck. She has talked about Big Buck for months. She has even asked Santa for Big Buck—numero uno on her Christmas list. "If Santa brings me Big Buck, Mama, I will hold my hand out. Like this. See? He will sniff it. And he will say 'neeeiiiggghhh.' Then we will be best buddies."

Imagine, maybe, the instant acceptance of baby when baby delivers Big Buck shortly after delivering herself or himself. For you, Big Sis, a good-faith gift, an "I am not here to steal your thunder, I just want to be a part of the family" gift.

Some call it the "terrible twos"; I call it the exploration of separation and independence. Big Sis has been wielding hers. Applying the idea that her thoughts are just as relevant to our family as mine or Wade's, Big Sis—who gave to herself that handle—equally gave to the bump the moniker "Julian." Where the name "Julian" came from, I do not know, and she has not disclosed. But it stuck.

She's gonna love it, Julian! I gleam, even in the darkness of the bedroom, envisioning the look on her face when Big Buck makes his grand entrance *before* Christmas.

I do believe Julian agrees, as another gentle yet electric squeeze wraps around my lower back.

With that, I figure I should softly sound the alarm. I tiptoe from the bedroom and down the hallway, pausing just before the living room, my eyes peeking around the corner.

There he is. His eyes model well-earned crinkles, only heightening his allure. His deep indulgent laugh fills up the space. He enjoys a little Saturday Night Live and a little Saturday Night Libation. His last night as a father to one, and he doesn't even know it...yet.

# Sleep...While You Can

WADE SPOTS ME. WELL, TECHNICALLY, HE SPOTS THE BUMP AS IT ROUNDS THE corner before I do.

"Couldn't sleep, huh," he says.

Not even midnight, I know he assumes my witching hour is showing off, a few hours ahead of schedule. In the first and second trimesters, the witching hour was spent emptying an instant-refill bladder and diverting nausea with a protein-packed snack, reading, and channel surfing. The nausea, akin to television commercials, apparently did not get the memo that it was overplayed. The third trimester witching hour, with its growing pains, includes the habits of the first and second, as well as relieving exercises, such as squatting and stretching with the assistance of the birthing hammock.

Shrewdly, Wade reaches one arm out to me—an invitation—while the other arm slides the remote to the far side of the end table. He finds my channel surfing more nauseating than the commercials. I chuckle, eyeballing the remote. To which he doubles down with a playful Clint Eastwood squint. Okay, fine. He had it first. That is the deal.

I'm not here to stay, at any rate. I'm headed back to bed. "You might want to get some rest, too," I tell him.

"Huh?" His eyes dart from the TV to mine, catching my drift. The only person in this house who has a bedtime curfew is the soon-to-be three-year-old already asleep.

I nod, raking my bottom lip through my teeth once more. It works. Tears of joy trapped, my voice can speak freely. "Something is happening, babe. I can feel it in my lower back."

"Oh...shit," he stammers mid sip. "Now? It's happening now?" Actions matching scattered thoughts, he clicks off the TV, springs up from couch, darts toward the kitchen, and pours the rest of his wine down the sink.

I laugh, in my own excitement at his overzealousness. "It's okay, babe. Breathe. Nothing is going to happen 'now.'"

"What can I do?" He chugs a glass of water and then chugs another, as if they could cancel each other out—two glasses of water neutralize two glasses of wine!

"Sleep."

"Sleep?!" Consternation flickers in his bugged-out eyes. If I had to guess, he has a shoulder nag, too. And much like mine, his yells. Sleep! Are you crazy! Who sleeps at a time like this! Shouldn't we be doing something!

"Yes, sleep." I am still full of giggles, nothing new in his company. "Sleep…while you can. It's gonna be a while."

"How do you know?"

"The 'squeezes,' babe. I only felt a couple. They're intermittent and far apart. At least thirty minutes apart…early, early labor. If this one is anything like Mila, it's gonna be a while. Which is good. We can sleep tonight, labor tomorrow." I state the perfect scenario out loud, maybe attempting to speak it into existence.

"Oooh, babe!" He whisper-shouts, dropping to his knees, hands caressing and lips pressing to the bump. "You hear that, Julian. Soon, my boy…or girl." His hesitation is spurred by intuition peppered in doubt. His gut tells him Julian is a boy. That must mean Julian is a girl. "You take it easy on Mama," he adds the gentle advisory, *soon* calling to his attention that *it* is about to get real.

The egg and sperm have come full circle.

Julian, wee babe, made of muscle and bone and connective tissue—half of Daddy's DNA tucked into the nuclei of cells that built the body that powers the muscle and bone and connective tissue—must pass through Mama's muscle and bone and connective tissue.

Not only a rite of passage but a literal passage, and a passing of genes from one generation to the next.

Oooh, I can see it! I am beginning to feel it. It is almost tangible. It is happening. Baby is almost here. Wade is right. Sleep? Who *could* sleep at a time like this?

Cart, get back behind the horse! The ol' nag barks at my anticipation. *Laborious* journey ahead! Go! To! Bed!

Strange, the ol' gal making her presence known at the start, when I would not hear from her again until it was time to push.

# Wonder Midwife

I WAS ABLE TO SLEEP FOR A FEW HOURS BEFORE THE LOWER BACK SQUEEZES required any soothing. More than the discomfort, the comfort of knowing that we would soon meet baby right here in our home was what kept me roused. Afforded a second chance at birth, so to speak, was almost more buoyancy than I could contain.

Whilst my restlessness was unlikely to wake Wade or Mila, as evidenced by the sleepy hum of their breathy and melodic Darth Vader duet, I thought myself considerate in relocating to the living room.

In doing so, I passed by the guest bedroom where Mom was catching a few z's of her own. She had flown in for the birth, and to care for Mila during the birth, and to help us transition from parents of one to parents of two. Although technically even, we would find ourselves outnumbered. I could wake Mom. She wouldn't mind. She wouldn't send me back to bed either. She would stay up with me. Then the sun would rise, and we would feel like two teenaged girls at a slumber party who wished we would have sacrificed our bras to the freezer and gone our butts to bed.

2:30 AM—the numbers emboldened themselves in cobalt blue from the cable box as I meandered my way back to the living room.

The universe. Yep, it was strutting its stuff again.

My children, the symmetry, the *oneness*. One was conceived one month after and one day before the other in a different year. One was born one month before and one day after the other in a different year. They weighed the same at birth, each with two ones in the ounce measure 11. The times at which they were born represent a difference of 1:11—one hour and eleven minutes. Mila was born to Willie's *Blue Eyes Crying in the Rain*, and it was cause for goosebumps when it, too, played on radio KVET 98.1 as we met Julian for the first time via ultrasound.

2:30 AM—that was the time when I lost my mucus plug with Mila. That was the time I went against instinct. The time I wanted to stay home and rest. The time I wanted to give things a chance to start naturally. The time I didn't.

Not this time.

I casually texted Genevieve, giving her a heads-up that things were slowly but surely shaping up, so she would not be surprised if her Sunday did not go quite as planned.

She actually texted back…at 2:30 in the morning…a Sunday morning.

I couldn't help but wonder, was she some kind of Wonder Midwife? You know, like Wonder Woman, ready and willing to answer the call whenever it comes?

As a nurse in postpartum, if I paged a doctor at 2:30 on a Sunday morning—after first being triaged through an answering service—and if the doctor felt as though my call required a return call, then…it better be good. Worthy of a wake-up call good.

2:30 AM

*Hi Genevieve. Just wanted you to know something is starting here. No big deal, some lower back pressure. Nothing active or regular. I'll update you tomorrow morning.*
SEND

I assumed that, like my phone, her phone was at the bottom of a purse or in the console of a vehicle, anywhere other than on her person when she wants to use it. I assumed she would get the message at a decent Sunday morning hour, and either I would have updated her if need be, or she would then get back to me. I did not mean to wake her. The nurse in me knew full well that my status was not worthy of a wake-up call.

2:33 AM

*Hi Brooklyn. How exciting! Can you tell me how far apart you're feeling the lower back pressure?*
RECEIVED

I jolted a bit in the recliner at the buzzing of the phone on the end table. Seriously? She's awake? Or she woke to text me back? I did not know which possibility impressed or embarrassed me more.

2:36 AM
*30-60 minutes apart, very intermittent. Just kind of achy and waking me here and there. The excitement is keeping me up more than the discomfort...lol. Sorry to text you at this hour.*
SEND

2:39 AM
*Don't be sorry. That's what I'm here for. And don't hesitate to text or call if you need me. Otherwise I'll talk to you in a few hours. It is exciting! But please try and rest while you can.*
RECEIVED

So I spent a couple of hours in the recliner, keeping in mind that my position may have much to do with baby's, especially so close to active labor. Although reclining, the recliner seemed supportive with its thirty-degree incline, providing a small assist via gravity. I was conscious of maintaining left-side lying position, where I collaboratively used a heating pad wrapped around my side—half of it warming my back and the other half warming my abdomen—hoping to keep baby's back and bottom in anterior position. The combination was helpful in providing periods of sleep.

In those other moments of temporary waking, as those once isolated lower back squeezes gained ground in wrapping their tentacles around my flanks and causing a crampy sensation in my uterus, I meditatively prepared.

Uh-huh, there you are, I thought to myself.

My mind found diversion from the twinge by directing its focus to the child who would go through this labor with me. Feel that, baby? We can handle that. We got this. Feel with me. Breathe with me. You and me, kid. Trust, surrender, accept. Now rest with me, dream with me of our meeting.

It must have registered on some psychosomatic level. I climbed back in bed with Wade and beside Mila around 5:30, and we all slept in until 7:30.

# Push That Baby Out

FOOD! I THOUGHT. GET IT IN WHILE YOU CAN.

Pain *is* nauseating.

A safe bet that my last meal until meeting baby would be breakfast, morning activity spurred more regular and assertive contractions.

By 9:30, I empathized with the fresh-squeezed orange juice I made and knocked back, along with a substantial and protein-rich feast. Once 30-60 minutes apart, my ambiguous and episodic "squeezes" had become clear and present contractions. No longer confined to my lower back and no longer simply crampy, the myometrium—middle layer and smooth muscle—of my uterus was full of intention, demanding my undivided attention for half a minute or so every three to ten minutes.

Everything the uterus did to shore up pregnancy would now have to be reversed. The myometrium that expanded in pregnancy, allowing babe the space to bloom, would have to contract in labor. The cervix, technically a part of the uterus, that closed and grew thick—a fortress—holding in and protecting babe, would have to thin/efface and open/dilate in labor. And the only way the uterus was going to pull off this about-face was through uniform contractions, steadfast intervals of shortening and tightening and flexing.

After seven hours of toying with the game plan, it appeared to be game-on for my uterus.

I could not help but think of my first birth experience. How I was induced because "nothing was happening." Because my water had trickled and regular contractions had not ensued. But the back squeezes were there. Just like they are here...intermittent and light. Then, literally overnight, it was go time. Seemingly instantaneous, a switch flipped. I will never know if the natural pattern would have progressed as such with Mila. Although I—like the old brain—just know it would have.

And we all know what they say about spilled milk, so I seized the moment and made a big to-do about the spectacular child I somehow won the favor of calling mine, regardless of how she got here.

She and "Grandma Glory" were headed to church, a perfect Sunday morning diversion while labor got underway. She picked out her clothes, coordinating them around boots, as any horse-loving cowgirl would.

We took our sweet time dressing her and fixing her hair, the last time we would do so as parents to one. As she sat on the vanity top, her boot-laden legs wriggling and wrapping around my thighs, she hugged and poked and stroked the bump, commenting how Julian "popped" my belly button "right out."

A nice segue to explain that it was, in fact, almost time to meet Julian.

"Today's a special day, baby, did you know that?" Daddy prefaced.

"Yes, because Grandma Glory's here." To be a grandparent! Wade and I are chopped liver—no offense to the powerhouse organ meat—in comparison. "And she's taking me to 'God's Castle.'"

"Uh-huh," I agreed. "And…Miss Genevieve's coming to spend some time with us today."

"Is she going to bring her *steff*oscope?"

"Yes, I bet she will have her *steth*oscope in tow. And Miss Katie, too."

"We're gonna have a pool in our dining room, baby!" Wade knew the birthing tub would be a subject of discussion eventually, so he prefaced that, too.

"A pool? Ooh, I'm sooo excited!" She fed off his energy before reality set in. "Buuut, but, but, I just wanna sit on the steps." We had hit some sort of fear wall, our cautious tot becoming altogether risk-averse—clinging to shoulders in the center of the pool last summer, but out there and facing fear nonetheless, to clinging to the edge this summer. Only to be independently treading water with the assistance of a noodle the next summer!

"This pool doesn't have steps, darlin'. It's called a *birthing* pool." My brows upraised with the clarification and with a contraction.

"Mmmhhh..." I groaned, rocking my hips from side to side and bracing my weight on the vanity top.

"The *birth* of the *baby*?" Her mind worked, putting it together.

"Yes, very good, honey," Wade encouraged her, allowing me to catch my breath. "We might get to meet Julian today. Would you like that?"

"Uh-huh. I will love him and hug him and tell him 'I'm Big Sis.' Aaand, and, and, I will play with him. But..." up came the index finger, "he can't have my bucks. No, sir."

"No worries, my girl..." I kissed the flesh between her brows, relieving the concerned furrow there. "Julian won't be playing with anything for some time. And you know that Julian might be a *she*, don't you?"

Accompanied with an appropriate bearing down, she said, "You have to puuush that baby out, like Blondie did Spirit in the sweet green grass." Then she neighed and whinnied, her nose nuzzling Julian.

I chuckled, before another "Mmmhhh...," wondering if she thought "he" was also a horse.

In the movie, Spirit's mother's name is Esperanza, but Mila refers to her as "Blondie," which is actually quite fitting, considering her palomino breed. As the movie opens, we meet Spirit shortly after Blondie wanders off alone to birth him in the tall grass. I love that the movie included this scene, a teaching theme that perfectly fit our life at the moment.

Of course, it is age appropriate. There is some neighing and whinnying and a look of despair, or determination, right before Spirit emerges behind Blondie who is lying/laboring on her side in a bed of grass. I was thankful Spirit didn't come by stork. Or that the vet didn't deliver him. And he actually suckled—sporting a cute milk mustache—moments after getting his wobbly legs under him, another nice bullet point for Big Sis.

The movie provided her first taking in of birth. She was naturally curious. And naturally, home birth books for tots were few and far between. So we ended up supplementing with a lot of explanation.

She even nosed in on watching birthing videos with me, out-gritting her daddy who could not bring himself to stomach them. The sounds of laboring women and birthed babes proved to be more than she could resist.

"Why is she making that noise? What's gonna happen, Mama?"

"She's laboring, baby, and labor *is* hard work. She's trying to puuush a baby out. A baby like Julian. We'll have to do that, too, puuush this baby out."

"Wonder if Mama will make noises like that?" Wade chided, his nose poked into his phone, checking fantasy football scores and avoiding any kind of a peek at our birthing video.

I ignored him, because I couldn't think of a comeback, and continued on with Mila, "You can watch, love, but don't feel like you have to. If it scares you, don't watch."

She answered my concern with more curiosity. As baby emerged, she cooed, "Ohhh, look at that baby. He's so cute." Again with *he*. "But why does he have food all over him?"

"Food?" Wade queried, daring to look up from his phone.

Jesus, Mary, and Joseph! He won't watch the birthing videos and he thinks food is a viable option as to what baby will be covered in upon birth? What kind of labor coach is he going to be?

"Vernix and blood," I deadpanned to Wade, before explaining to Mila, "you see that white cheesy-looking stuff? It helps protect baby's skin and keeps baby warm. It's called vernix caseosa."

"Like tapioca?" she asked.

"Close enough," I said, with a chuckle. "And there is a little blood…"

"Like a boo-boo, does it hurt that baby?"

"Not really like a boo-boo, and, well, I don't know if it hurts that baby. That's a really good question that no one has been able to answer with certainty. But, the baby isn't bleeding. The blood comes from baby's mama, from her uterus and cervix and vagina…"

"I, I, I have a 'gina.' But no one can touch it. I would say 'stop!'"

"Attagirl!" Wade encouraged her boundary.

"Is that baby gonna drown?" Back to the birthing video, just like that.

"No, darlin', that baby is not going to drown. Its mama had it in a birthing tub, that's all. And remember, that baby lived in water…amniotic fluid…in its mama's uterus. Just like you did, when I grew you in mine."

"Why is that baby crying?"

"It's trying out its lungs, filling them with air. You see, when baby was in that amniotic fluid in mama's uterus, mama basically breathed for baby. Now that baby is born, baby breathes for itself. You just witnessed that baby take its first breath. Pretty magical, huh."

"What is that rope?"

"You know," I coaxed, tickling her belly button, "you were attached to Mama by the…?"

"*Lum*bilical cord!"

"*Um*bilical cord, yes!" High five.

"After Julian is born, you and Daddy could cut the umbilical cord, if you want to." I did not look in Wade's direction, but only assumed he wrinkled up his nose, as averse to the idea as witnessing anything "down there."

"With *twizzers*?"

"Well, yeah, a special kind of *scissors*."

"Will Julian cry?"

"Cutting the umbilical cord won't hurt Julian because there aren't any nerves in it."

"But will he cry? When he comes out? Like that baby?"

I imagined Julian would cry. Any birth I witnessed, baby cried or was stimulated to, directly, to clear fluid from the airway. So I said, "Julian probably will cry, darlin'. Remember, you cried when you were born. It has to be an emotional journey, not to mention the change in habitat. And babies can't talk, right. So their cry is kind of like their communication to get what they need…arms to hold them and full bellies." My fingertips stroked her full belly, relying on the featherlight touch to bring its usual and instant relief, a zoning out.

But like any of us who cannot let go of our child's cry until it stops, she was not letting go of the mere thought of the start of Julian's.

"Will Julian cry?" she must have asked every time we watched a birthing video.

# Now

With Mila and Grandma Glory off to "God's Castle" by 10:00 AM, I got into the zone.

First things first, every clock in the house was set to now. With pre-made index cards clipped to size and inscribed by hand, I taped over any numeric and measurable version of time. The only time there ever truly is—N:OW (now o'clock).

We were on labor time. As *Birthing From Within* said, "Labor has its own clock."

On the clock, posthaste, with our hospital birth before labor even began, I did not want to see a clock. Do not tell me what time it is. If I ask, tell me it is now.

No clock, no sense of time, was beyond encouraging, a true labor-saver. Any labor is long enough. But the labor, like the pot, that is not watched seemed quicker to *boil*, shorter than it actually was. And it would be, a third of the time of our first birth. One-third the time in labor? One-third the time to complete dilation? That is huge. That is the difference between mental and physical exhaustion and having the energy left to push.

My last keeping of time on labor day was 9:48, 9:52, 9:54, 9:57, 10:00, and 10:03. Those times, requested by Genevieve and recorded on the back of page three of my Chant Sheet, represented the minutes between contractions.

Genevieve checked in earlier that morning, as she said she would. A follow-up to the initial checking in, I was to time contractions for fifteen minutes. In retrospect, I am so thankful she had me do this. Those times represent the only definitive record of time I have for labor, until the time of birth, of course. A stroke of serendipity, those times are a permanent part of my souvenir Chant Sheet, the only paper on which I could think to write as I was rehearsing it until I could no longer focus on it.

Soon after I reported the contraction intervals via text, Genevieve called. I could talk to her at this point without losing much breath or concentration. Although I did notice my own voice slipping into a contralto register, that tone at the furthest end of the breastbone just above the diaphragm. "Chesty" and introverted, it, like my mind, was in search of our solar plexus—the center of myself—where energy, power, emotional stability can be found.

If Genevieve took my ability to talk through contractions the same as I—an indication of early labor but not active labor—she wasn't in a hurry. I adored this about her, this sense, feel, intuition, experience. She just knew when to let me be and when to attend. While she is the first to say she "hopes she is a good midwife but makes mistakes and suffers with indecision sometimes about the right path to take," her pacing with this drawing back/stepping in was spot-on. I appreciated being able to labor as though she was not there even though she was. It felt more secure than any safety net I may have had in the hospital.

It was perfect, Wade and I in early labor together, alone. We needed that. To prepare ourselves and to prepare each other.

As our playlist crooned from the portable wireless speaker, we paced and prepared, singing along here and there. Wade transported the dining room table somewhere, I cannot recall, to make room for Genevieve's portable birthing tub. I gathered the birthing kit and a few other recommended supplies so that they would be accessible in one place for my midwife and her apprentice. Wade prepped the garden hose and the kitchen faucet adapters needed to fill the birthing tub. I checked the spare bedroom closet one last time for Julian's birth gift to Big Sis. Yes, Big Buck is there, wrapped and ready.

"This is it, babe!" Wade whisper-yelled, for the fifth time, his sexy little smile beaming with wonder.

I leaned into his conveniently-timed embrace, another exhaled "Mmmhhh..." accompanied the wringing of my uterus.

"What can I do?" he asked.

"You're doing it, babe. Just be here." My sappy smile, vanishing in an instant, was replaced by an imminent and nauseating kind of "Mmmhhh..."

I jetted for the bathroom. Breathe, stay calm, open the diaphragm, cold cloth on back of neck, I chanted internally, assembling one and staving off the heave.

Wade showed up at the door with a stainless steel bowl. I did not point out that it was my preferred bowl for whipping cream. No, I did not. I took it and thanked my thoughtful husband, my thoughtful birth partner.

To which he brandished his phone and said, "Say cheese, before you start puking."

To which I laughed and forgot I had to retch. Thank you again, I guess?

I did not appreciate the picture at the time, but, once more in retrospect, I love that he took it. It is the only picture of our labor. Requiring conscious effort, both of us disinclined to the distraction, we fail to capture all of the still memories we should. But that one shot says it all. My eyes, my expression, say it all. I have never seen myself like that. So in my body and on my way to a far-off land—Laborland.

The nausea said to me that it was time to curb the excitement about the initiation of labor and get on to the work of labor.

Remember the brain stem? It is where the "old brain" aka the "reptilian brain," in this particular case the "birthing brain," resides. You got it. *It* controls vomiting, too. Any basic involuntary bodily function is controlled by the brain stem, the body's "autopilot."

Doing its duty, the old brain protects. Vomiting is protection. If you feel about throwing up the way most of us do, you may need a moment to process that. So I say again, vomiting is protection—a body's way to rid itself of harmful foods and toxins.

Similar to a chain reaction, pain triggers the autonomic nervous system, which triggers hyperactivity in the brain, which triggers a spike in hormones aiming to correct/maintain homeostasis, which results in a feeling of sickness/nausea.

In other words, there is too much going on at one time. Too much going on at one time can be noxious, toxic, representative of a "toxin" to the nervous system, to the body, to the brain.

My thinking brain could not process all of it—pain, anticipation, preparation, pacing, music, smiling for the camera—neither accurately nor logically. My body, regulated by the old brain, naturally and instinctively wanted to compensate and protect itself/me from all of it...by virtue of losing my cookies.

In essence, that first wave of nausea said to me that labor was shaping up, a foghorn that my birthing brain is available. All I had to do was reach out to it.

My birthing brain, like my mother used to call to me at summer sundown, was saying "You've played enough. Get in here. Now!"

My birthing brain needed my presence to know that I/we were safe from danger. That we were safe from all of the external *it*, so that it could exclusively focus on the task at hand: birthing.

I could ignore my birthing brain, staying logical and thinking, where I could also fear and fail and puke. Or I could find my birthing brain, coexist with it, surrender myself to it, where it could do what it has done for pregnant women through the ages—busy itself with my survival and reproductive success.

"No more pictures," I said to Wade, withdrawing to the living room.

He dutifully clutched my whipping bowl, making sure it was within my reach. And I almost escaped an entire labor without needing it...almost.

# She's Got The Look

*Trust. Surrender. Accept. Your body knows how to do this.*

Again and again, the ingrained mantra was chanted in my mind. In no hurry, the cloud-like letters, inducing not only words but my birthing spirit, came and went. Drifting in and out, they were full of persuasion, slow enough for me to digest. The old brain and I were syncing.

Disengaging from mindfulness, I was able to honor my body. In that instinctual body, I crawled around on the floor. I squatted with the support of the birthing hammock. I sat on the birthing ball, rocking my pelvis from side to side and front to back. I knelt in front of the couch, elbows propped upon it, as if praying. Maybe I was. When all of this seemed too much, I tucked my knees beneath me and tucked my forehead to the floor, retreating into myself in Child's Pose.

Everything stationed in the living room, each move was but a crawl away. Looking back, I am surprised I wasn't more mobile.

I envisioned being upright, pacing and walking and leaning on Wade, something, anything that would hold me. All of this seemed feasible and ideal for me, a generally active person. Wouldn't I labor best actively?

Genevieve would actually have to remind me throughout labor that it was time to stand and move, change it up, let gravity help.

The only thing I can attribute my inactivity to would be a conscious desire to have the stamina required to birth at home. I told myself if I ended up birthing at the hospital, it would not be due to fatigue. Having experienced a rather lengthy first labor, I planned on a lengthy second labor. Wasteful with the rest between contractions in my first—on my feet pacing and jouncing, filled with fear and fight, psyching myself up for the next contraction, as if it were some sort of race to be won or weight to be pressed—I would *not* make the same mistake in my second.

Conserve. Conserve. Conserve…energy. The credo was embedded in every laboring action.

Eyes closed, body relaxed, introverted into oblivion, I rested between contractions.

And it worked smashingly.

Although it did not exactly facilitate the fantasy labor I might have envisioned. Okay, yeah, I envisioned it; there was no "might" about it. Wade and I would love and laugh our way through labor. We would manage each contraction and spend the time between giving and receiving love and reminiscence, a recount of how our family started.

"Remember the first time you struck up conversation in the gym, using my Terrible Towel as the segue?" I would say. "One minute, my sweaty face was disguised behind it. Only to let it fall, and there you were. When you said 'So, you're a Steelers fan?' I would have said something like 'What was your first clue?' But I was too busy picking my jaw up off the floor, just looking at you."

"It wasn't my best opening line, I'll admit, but I had to say something. You were finally accessible, doing push-ups right beside me," he would say. "Straight on military push-ups...and a lot of 'em. That's when I knew...this girl ain't playing around. I noticed you long before that, though. I told my friend, I said, 'Dude, there's this girl at my gym...' 'Talk to her, bro...' he said. It just took me a while to find my confidence."

"Who needs confidence with your eyes? So light, upswept lashes so dark, and the warmth in them, mmh...that's the first thing I noticed about you."

"You have great eyes, too, but I'd be lying if I said that's the first thing I noticed about you." Wade would laugh and I would laugh because he had already told me that it was my keister. No, he did not say "keister." He said, "You've got a great ass."

"You may not be much of a romantic, but you're such a good man," I would swoon, leaning my forehead into his at the start of another contraction.

"You're a better woman," he would swoon back, his confidence in me lifting my own in our birth.

And blah romantic blah reminiscent blah...

Yeah, none of that happened. I was on another plane most of my labor, I can't even remember if I told him I loved him or thanked him, unfortunately.

I knew he was there. My eyes closed and focused inward, I could feel him—a gentle hand on my back, cool breath on my face, his presence when there was no contact at all. For every contraction, every rest, he was there, so patient and compassionate. I don't know how he did it, had the wherewithal to endure something that wasn't even happening to him physically. The patience and sympathy that must have taken. And he said the same to me, that he didn't know how I did it, labored and birthed naturally. He thinks he would have wanted the epidural!

Those first hours of active labor, when contractions were most easily managed, remain my most dreamlike hours in birth. I know that was me. I was there, in that body and laboring. But I am hard-pressed to recall much of it. Even as I was going through it, it was strange, unearthly. Is this me? Am I here?

I remember when Genevieve first arrived, but I cannot recall if her apprentice Katie was with her then. Wade welcomed Genevieve and she sized me up with one glance, saying, "Oh, yeah...she's got the look."

In retrospect, I surmise "the look" is some "birth bearing," some "mien of a birthing woman"—a specific way of moving, a particular kind of appearance or manner only birthing women exhibit. And I surmise that midwives are astute in recognizing the look because they have seen it in naturally laboring women and rely on it more than technology in assessing the woman.

At the time, I just remember thinking, I have the look? *Yes*, I do. It was encouraging. It registered highly enough with me to recall it at a time when there wasn't much I recalled, period. It said to me that we were on the right track. Laborland, here we come!

I am quite certain Genevieve did a cervical check to get a baseline, because I can see myself lying on the living room floor, and I think I was dilated three centimeters. Still much laboring to be done. I feel like Katie had to be there because I think I recall Genevieve saying "they" would like to go get some lunch if I was okay with "them" leaving.

I was okay with that. They could do nothing for me at that point. Again, I appreciated the privacy.

In the meantime, Mila and Grandma Glory came in from God's Castle and left again to go to the playground. My mother was such a helpful sport in keeping Mila happily occupied. We couldn't have done it without her.

I do not remember them coming back from church. I do not remember them changing from church clothes to play clothes. I do not remember them leaving for the playground.

"Remember when you were pushing that baby out, and your head was like this on the couch," Mila said a few weeks later as we cuddled on the couch, where she acted out for me a forward-kneeling rest between contractions.

"You were there with me?" I asked.

"Yeah, after God's Castle. Were you sleeping?"

"I was resting, baby, between contractions." Why can't I recollect that? My child being there with me, being there for me.

I also have no recollection of Genevieve and Katie coming back from lunch, although I know they did. I can see both of them on the living room couch, one with a tablet and one knitting. Yet if you required me to tell you which one was doing what, I am not certain I could.

I do not remember Wade updating me on the Steelers game, but he says he did, and that I had asked him the score.

I cannot recall when or how the portable birthing tub got inflated. Don't you think I would remember the sound of the air pump? But I distinctly remember the sound of water filling it and how much I looked forward to getting into that water.

Remember when you were a kid and your mom made cookies and she pulled that first batch from the oven? Wherever you were, whatever you were playing, you could sense it—the aroma pulling you by the olfactory, feet following nose, until you were standing guard, and salivating, over that tray of cookies. You knew you were allowed one, as soon as they would not melt the skin off the roof of your mouth. Did anything ever take longer than for that first batch of cookies to cool down?

That is how I felt about the filling of the birthing tub.

The drawing of that water drew me out of the living room and into the dining room. It lured my birthing bones the way my mother's cookies lured my adolescent appetite. Crawling-squatting-forward-leaning guard around it as it filled, if muscles could salivate mine would have anticipating the relief they would feel submerged in warm water.

The same as inspiring me with a simple but impactful "she's got the look," I clearly recall the equally motivating and meaningful words Genevieve chose to say to me right before I got into the birthing tub. Another simple one-liner that this laboring woman, otherwise preoccupied, could retain.

"You've earned this time in the tub," she said.

Earned? *Yes*, I had.

Although Genevieve would likely not consider herself a beacon but rather a "cheerleader," she was a guiding light for me. A ray of energy that illuminated peacefulness and patience, she emitted both naturally.

I have come a long way in accepting and understanding that fast does not equate to efficient. But that still does not stop my natural energy from being in quest of, and motivated by, the endgame. That most thrilling part when all of the effort begins to take shape, when the goal has never been closer, when the end is intensely palpable. Absolutely, I get off on that.

Looking back, it is plain to see that in my hospital birth when given impatience, my eagerness did me no favors in saying, okay, I'll see that and raise you. In my home birth, I would learn that the course on which I arrive and the energy with which I arrive to the endgame makes all the difference. I would also learn that in natural birth there are no shortcuts to that most rewarding and anticipatory part: there are no shortcuts to the endgame.

Genevieve's energy, from her tone of voice and its cadence to her manner and its rhythm, was purposeful but calm, carrying out but in no hurry. I needed that.

And although Genevieve would say "the greatest success of any birth is the birthing woman, her determination, her trust, her attitude," I am once more reminded of Robbie Davis-Floyd's position: "I have long believed and have stated many times in my oral presentations that the most important determinants of the outcome of a woman's birth are the attitudes and ideology of her primary caregiver(s)."

# Laborland

FOR A RELATIVELY INACTIVE LABORING WOMAN, I LET NO DUST SETTLE WHEN the birthing tub was filled.

Leggings, panties, bra—gone!

Ahhh…

Although I read about, and had even seen in some of those birthing videos, women birthing completely naked, I guess I never thought to consider *would I*? At that point in my labor, I did not consider it either. What was covered or uncovered, and whoever saw whatever, mattered not to me one iota.

That birthing tub was essential, a must-have. A birthing tub that I instinctively wanted in my hospital birth, but was not accommodated, would be accommodated at no extra charge, requiring extra effort in transporting and maintaining, in our home birth. The effort and maintenance were not wasted.

That birthing tub was as blissful as it could get for this laboring woman.

Contractions were steadily gaining in force, wearing down my psyche, requiring more energy to stay calm and relax through. The second my body submerged into that tub, not only did it feel like a huge weight released, it also allowed me to recapture some strength. Okay, yes, I can manage this.

Providing some pleasure with the pain, I could hear my own groans morphing into moans. Here comes another squeeze! Ohhh, Jesus, this hurts. But this water, ahhh. Thank you, Lord, for this water.

Rest between contractions in the water was unparalleled. Straight-up sleep, as if I were knock-knock-nobody's-home gone, unreachable, the only thing capable of pulling me out of the slumber was a recurring contraction. Even those were foggy. A moan, an exhale, maybe a contortion of the hips and pelvis, but my eyes and my mind were closed unto themselves.

In that birthing tub, I found Laborland.

Ina May Gaskin said, "If a woman doesn't look like a goddess during labor, then someone isn't treating her right."

I would surmise the odds of my looking like a goddess during labor were as plausible as pigs flying, regardless of the exceptional treatment I was receiving, but I sure felt like a goddess in that water.

Whatever shift my hormones and endorphins were experiencing, the Laborland effect, I see why it is said that natural labor can provide natural pain relief unrivaled by man-made drugs. That rest between contractions still befuddles me. I do not rest that deeply per my usual sleep routine, devoid of labor and pain, taking longer than the time between contractions to fall asleep and next to nothing to wake me. The capability to fall in and out at such short intervals, utterly slumberous, had to be some untapped force, somewhere inside myself I have never been. A secret labor euphoria. A high I will never attain again. Somewhere inside myself I will never go again…unless there is another natural labor in my future.

The amnesia of it all. Not that we forget the pain of childbirth, but it doesn't seem nearly as disagreeable in hindsight. The amnesia of laboring itself. That has to be hormones and endorphins, some protective "old brain/knowing body" natural affect, right?

Why else can't I recall Mila telling me that she loved me while I was laboring. I should remember that. I *would* remember that in any other circumstance, free from the influence of laboring hormones and endorphins.

"Do you remember when you were in that water, Mama, before you pushed that baby out?" Mila asked.

"Yes, I do. Do you remember that?" I asked back, unaware if she did.

She nodded. "Grandma Glory and I came home from the playground. And I said 'I love you, Mama.'" She grinned sheepishly, proud of her sweet little loving self.

"You said that to me? When I was in the birthing tub?" I quizzed myself more than her, feeling a bit a bad mom that I could not recall such a tender moment. "What did I say when you told me you loved me?" Please, let me have returned her affection.

"You said 'I love you more.'" She grinned even more sheepishly, a toddler's need for love always a skosh more than the need to give it.

I squeezed her to me, and over her shoulder, the breath I held hostage fluttered from my lips like air from a balloon. Bad mom forgiven.

Lucidity escaped me in Laborland.

I have flashes of music from the playlist, which is nothing to brag about seeing how the speaker was an arm's reach from my ears. I recall someone singing along to an Eagles song. I think it was Katie, and I think it was *Take It Easy*. I believe I recall hearing baby's heartbeat via Genevieve's waterproof Doppler. I remember being offered something to drink. I tried but not very well, either taking too much effort or altogether unappetizing.

I think it was shortly thereafter that Genevieve encouraged me up and out of the tub, fanning a bit of wind in my sails and directing high-knees walking up and down the hallway. It reminded me of what we called "z-sprints" in high school sports conditioning; no one wants to do them, but they do pay off.

Genevieve's instinct impeccable, again, I did not realize how lethargic I had become in the tub. If left to my own Laborland devices, I would have hunkered down in that thing like draft opponents during the Vietnam War: Hell no, we won't go!

Whilst birthing tubs have proven to be helpful, specifically in reducing the need/desire for epidural, too much of any good thing can backfire. It has also been proven that birthing tubs, specifically in early labor, can slow labor, make worse dehydration, and add to overall lethargy.

Yes, it was time to change things up—different position, different energy—doing so often persuading labor along.

Standing from the tub *was* rather shocking. The weight returned to my bones. The weight of contractions returned to my uterus. Abruptly cold and aware, I imagine I felt like a newborn babe. Put me back in!

Genevieve and Katie toweled me off. Wade helped me into a cozy robe. And Maren Morris sang *My Church* from the portable speaker. The song, one of Mila's personal additions to the playlist, was enough to prompt me to ask where she and Mom were. Wade said they had come in from the playground and went back out for an adventure walk.

It was time for me to walk, too, get active.

I remember feeling happy, gleeful, a surge of energy on my feet. I attempted even to sing along with Maren, before realizing it took far too much energy. Another thing I envisioned is that I would sing/chant aloud far more than I actually did.

I focused, instead, on my slow and steady high-knees technique up and down the hallway. Wade followed and coached along, the peewee football coach in him finally getting a moment to shine. Yes, this part of laboring was in his wheelhouse. With each contraction, he was right there for me to turn to. While I latched my hands around his neck, he supported my weight. This helped tremendously in allowing gravity to assist in a full upright position; otherwise, I know my knees would have buckled beneath the burden.

My mind flashed back to that first peewee football game I watched him coach—the one where I realized my heart belonged to him, the one where those kiddos were leaning on his big ol' broad shoulders. Now I know why God gave them to him; not only to hold those sweet kiddos up but to hold me up, too, as I labored his child into the world.

After what I am guesstimating to be about forty-five minutes of the high-knees routine, I wanted to curse myself for getting into the birthing tub. You should have waited a little longer! It was so relieving that anything thereafter was going to be disappointing, harder to manage.

Yet I couldn't have been too upset with myself because I went right back into it.

Here I go, once more, unable to remember how or when or why, exactly, I got back into the tub. Weaseling likely played a role. I could not—did not want to—help myself. Like a toddler who enjoys bath time, I had one thing on my mind, and it was that water. To this day, my curiosity remains unquelled: What would it have been like to birth in the water?

Birthing in the tub *was* the fantasy—akin to laughing and loving our way through contractions, akin to being present when our firstborn told me that she loved me while laboring for our second born, akin to chanting/singing as a pain coping mechanism, yada yada "ideal birth" yada.

We all know that fantasy and actuality rarely link up, which is pretty fantastic because actuality routinely proves itself to be more interesting, definitely more educational.

Looking back, I doubt I would have tolerated the tub for pushing, anyhow. I wasn't together enough, serene enough. Wade would've had his work cut out for him in attempting to keep my head above water. Once I hit transition and pushing, which felt like a simultaneous occurrence, my birth warrior, beast, animal, whatever you want to call her, exerted herself. She, too, contrary to the fantasy, was nothing like I envisioned.

Flower child, yes, that was my vision. I would be peaceful, composed, cool. I would recognize the pain and handle it gracefully, releasing it from my body with a flowing exhale. My hair would be long and loose, cascading around laid-back shoulders, maybe a leather headband or bandana keeping it in place.

Right.

Only annoyed by it—heavy, hot, unruly—my hair was looped through itself in a sloppy bun atop my head. Move over flower child, here comes *Xena: Warrior Princess*, "Ayiyiiyiyiyiyi!" And it is time to get shit done.

"All the inhibitions and trappings of our social selves are peeled away as our bodies thrust and heave, vomit and grunt, cry and leak. The animal is there for everyone to see." —Susan Diamond, obstetrical nurse, doula, childbirth instructor

That quote resonated with me the instant I read it. Paraphrases of it made their way onto, and were earnestly memorized from, my Chant Sheet. Instinct knew better than reason or illusion my birth actuality.

As I catapulted from my back to all fours in the middle of our bed, that first urge to push so shocking and vivid, the sound catapulting itself from my gut and out of my mouth was even more shocking. I never heard a cry quite like that come from my body.

Eyes widening, knees tamping the mattress below, surely I looked like a terrified horse. My shallow breathing reminiscent of a snort, I expected I might actually neigh. But the sound that finally emitted itself from my sympathetic-charged nervous system via an instantly dry mouth and gritty vocal cords was no whinny. It was a moo...howl... roar?

Before I reared back and lunged at the wall, hands gripping into it as if climbing it were an option. I swear I thought I could.

I wanted to get hold of myself. But I couldn't. I was unavailable. Something, someone had taken over. And it took a few minutes to relinquish the urge to tame this untamable part of me. Who are you? What are you doing? And what the hell is that noise? A moo-howl-roar? A cow-wolf-bear?

Wolf, sure. Bear, alright. Cow? Maybe a breastfeeding omen of sorts, but my creative side would have opted for something a bit more majestic—say a horse...a mustang...even a terrified one.

Proof! That reality always asserts itself over fantasy, especially in Laborland.

# Rabbit Hole

I COULDN'T HAVE BEEN IN THE TUB VERY LONG THE SECOND TIME. I JUST remember thinking that I wanted to stay there indefinitely. But I needed to get out. It was time to get out.

Mom and Mila had come in for the evening. It was getting dark. They had to be hungry. And I didn't even consider making them dinner. Normally, I would make my child dinner. I would certainly make my mother a proper dinner, a thank you. A detail that kind of bothers me to this day. That in my labor I was bereft of the ability to think of anything other than laboring.

I migrated from the dining and living rooms to the bedroom. One, I wanted to give Mom and Mila space to relax and settle into a nighttime routine without worrying about disrupting me. Mom would consider that. Two, I did not want to be disrupted.

Hence, the cow—the moo of the moo-howl-roar—was perfect. Any animal, really, will usually seek privacy when birthing. Growing up on a dairy farm, I had some experience in animal birthing, cows specifically. Yet I just realized I never considered any of those the "first birth" I had ever witnessed. Hmm.

We were not sheltered from watching the mama cows labor and birth their calves. Maybe Mom thought it was a good lesson in reproduction…or eventually abstinence! We were allowed to observe, from a distance. With full understanding that you do not touch, make loud noises or sudden movements, invade their space, or otherwise disrupt the process.

I could not imagine tending to anyone else's needs or entertainment while tending to labor. A jack of all trades—master of none—and multitasking fool, labor and birth was a whole different animal.

Judging from the darkness that followed sundown through the bedroom window, I would say it may have been near six o'clock on this late fall evening.

That absence of light was symbolic of how I started to feel. Restless, not exactly doubtful but wondering, contractions harder and harder to manage. Could I keep this up?

Pressing, cramping, aching, burning, radiating, pulling, and spreading—to me contractions represented the pain that keeps on evolving. Likely a different *contraction cocktail* for every woman, the exact mix differing throughout labor, could it be the contractions do not want us to get bored.

I attempted to hearten myself with the fact that natural contractions felt more user-friendly than the induced/augmented contractions I experienced in my first birth. Although, maybe my babies' positions had something to do with that as well. It may stand to reason that labor, precisely back labor, with an OP positioned babe in my first birth was more insufferable than an optimal OA positioned babe in my second. It just seemed to me that induced contractions were more intense, more aggressive—very in-my-face—with little rest between from the get-go.

In hindsight, I would add that induced contractions felt out of sync with me, my body, my rhythm. I can only imagine it felt the same for Mila. Sans liberty to establish our natural rhythm and under the influence of inducing agents, she and I never got to experience that natural syncing. The miscommunication between hormones and feedback loops, brain and body, mama and baby that were ultimately caused by intervention only resulted in more intervention.

Those past hospital birthing interventions fueled present home birthing fortitude. Fortitude I would need in the face of mounting uncertainty.

Supposedly the restlessness and doubt and feeling of "Can I keep this up?" is perfectly normal in the transition phase. This shift primes the sympathetic nervous system, primes catecholamines, primes the mind and body to rise to the occasion, so to speak. This shift, because I was unprepared and under the clock and prematurely riddled with fight or flight in response to fear, happened too early in my first birth. There was no way to maintain such an adrenaline shift from kickoff. The early shift coupled with the induction and eventually the epidural only worked against the process, slowing labor to a crawl.

Attributable to preparation, being comfortably in my own space at home and an undisturbed process, this shift was impeccably timed in my second birth. Naturally arranged, my hormones were like the conductor; my body the orchestra. We had just come through our long drawn-out and steady score—early and active phases of labor. The conductor would eventually and seamlessly direct the orchestra into *accelerando*: a gradual increase in tempo. The stress of such tempo eliciting excitement and a healthy skosh of fear is nature's blueprint for the quintessential transition. The transition from laboring to birthing.

Yes, I was slowly and naturally leaving Laborland. The dreamlike state was wearing off; the narcoleptic rest was thinning.

I wanted to stand and move around, but I could not or simply did not. I wanted to lie down, and I did, but writhed restlessly. The contractions were slipping away from me, neither able to wrap my mind nor my pain preparation techniques around them. My breathing grew shallow and weak and worried.

Those groans once turned to moans in the birthing tub were now verging on pathetic pleas. Cold and shaky one minute, hot and sweaty the next. I had to pee or poop or puke; I couldn't tell which. I had to get comfortable, find my way back to center, find my way back to Laborland.

But I couldn't. Like *Alice in Wonderland*, I was in the rabbit hole.

Did I want a way out? Had I been in the hospital, an epidural would have been mighty tempting. This "bizarre and disorienting alternate reality"—otherwise known as Transition—where I started to feel susceptible, was about to get a bit more bizarre and disorienting. Before clarity and constancy in the form of "the urge to push" would shove me onward to birthing.

There was no turning back. There was only one way to get from Laborland to Birthland. And that was through Transition.

Laborland, Transition, and Birthland remind me of screenwriting where one could easily assign the "three-act structure" of Setup, Confrontation, and Resolution. Three distinct tones that I missed in my hospital birth where intervention, whether induction or cesarean, became the "event," muddying the Catalyst, Rising Action, and Climax. In our home birth, birth was the event, more riveting than any movie I ever witnessed.

Shortly after I retreated to the bedroom, Genevieve took to hydrating me. A great call on her part, as I had not been taking in much fluid at all by mouth. Another thing I did not expect, even water was hard to stomach in labor. She did not prescribe or order the IV fluids, but simply put it out there: "This is what I would like to do." I was willing and appreciated the choice. There is power in a choice, maybe power that somehow motivated me through that vulnerable time. A subtle "Yes, let's do that" choice that motivated a larger "Yes, let's do this" determination.

Genevieve made clear that we would not leave the IV in. It would be nothing cumbersome or irritating that I would have to deal with for any length of time while dealing with labor. She would place it, allow the fluids to infuse via gravity, then remove it immediately thereafter.

I liked that the fluids infused via gravity rather than the additional clumsiness and hum of a pump. Even more than that, I liked the comfort of my bed and my surroundings while the fluids infused via gravity.

I would estimate that it took twenty minutes per bag to infuse, so roughly forty minutes altogether. And I did feel a bit of an energy boost from the hydration, facilitating another pass at high knees around the bed.

On one of those passes, a trickle ran down my leg. Thinking maybe it was membranes rupturing, I was surprised at the color.

"Oh, a little blood?" I half said, half questioned.

"Oh, that's a good sign," Genevieve immediately soothed.

A good sign? *Yes*, it was.

Dilation was progressing, cervix ripening, my first "bloody show."

On that aforementioned dairy farm and when watching mama cows give birth, when a little blood would dribble from mama cow's bum—vagina, technically—my sisters and I would look at each other and wrinkle up our noses as if to say "What's that!" This usually happened near the end and when mama cow was restless and on her feet and pacing and "bawling," farmer talk for moo-crying. It wasn't long thereafter that the calf was born.

And it wouldn't be long thereafter that I would bear my own child. If I could just bear Transition. If I could bear the rabbit hole.

Upon my first and reassuring bloody show, Genevieve checked to see where we were. I remember, seven centimeters. My bag of waters was leading the way. In other words, the amniotic sac rather than baby's head was pressing on and dilating my cervix. She explained that we could continue on, uninterrupted, and the sac would eventually and fully dilate the cervix and/or break out of the way for baby's head to take over. Or we could break/rupture the sac.

This "artificial rupture of membranes" is done with an "amnihook" that resembles a plastic crochet hook. Passing through the vagina and cervix, the amnihook grabs a piece of the balloon-like sac, snags it and breaks it, where the fluid then leaks out. Breaking of waters is usually done to either augment or induce labor. In my case, the goal would be to augment labor, to help dilation along, as baby's head is usually more efficient than the sac in dilating the cervix.

Again, the choice was mine.

A flurry of things raced through my conscience: Rupturing membranes? But I want everything to be "natural." We're already at seven. It is natural. A little push can't hurt? But that—a little push—is what got us into trouble the first time. This is *not* the first time. This is Genevieve, who wouldn't have mentioned it if she thought it was going to impede anything. Her instincts have been true.

"Yes," my instinct spoke aloud, "let's try that."

The same with wondering how birthing in the tub would have actualized, I wonder how labor would have progressed without breaking waters. That's just me. As much as I believe "All who wander are not lost," I also believe "All who wonder are not confused," but curious, eager for the experience.

At the time, and in this birth, it seemed a potentially promising way out of or through the rabbit hole. Wherever it led or whatever it led to,

I had no clue, having never been there before. Having never made it that far in my first birth.

In my physical and mental state in the transition of my second birth, I was willing to test it out.

I didn't even consider would it or could it backfire? I had read about the pros and cons of artificial rupture of membranes. I knew that an artificial rupture before labor or in early labor carried the risk of more intervention. I knew that artificial rupture in active labor, and in transition specifically, almost always speeds up labor, but that some women felt it neither hindered nor progressed their births.

"Do what is right for you," I remember the widely shared advice from birth blogs and forums.

So I followed instinct.

And she didn't disappoint!

# Moo-Howl-Roar

AHHH, I MOANED INTERNALLY, OR MAYBE OUT LOUD.

The warmth of my waters was relaxing, not only on my skin but even relieving a bit of cervical-uterine-genitourinary pressure. I did not expect that. It was heavenly…for a moment.

The time between stripping membranes/breaking waters and the next contraction felt, well, like a nice break! Longer than any other time between active contractions, it felt abating, alleviating, maybe even thrilling…for a moment.

In the next moment, with the next contraction, I catapulted from flat on my back to all fours on my front with no recollection of how exactly I did so. Many a year since I engaged in gymnastics, not to mention that for the last three months of pregnancy any movement from a lying position required some rolling and purposeful momentum to change, I had to defy the laws of gravity or physics in how I got there. And there I was. There *we*—the cow-wolf-bear—were, letting loose our first mighty moo-howl-roar.

What in time is that! I wondered, before realizing it came from me, some untapped vocal rumpus.

If ever there was a time in labor when my proclivity for resting and saving energy dissolved, this was that time. No way could I have lay down or rested comfortably at this point, unless I had an epidural. If ever there was a time in labor when an epidural could have seemed a fantastically great idea, this was that time. If ever there was a time in labor when I wanted out, *this was that time.*

You put your hand on something hot, too hot, it hurts, what do you do? You pull it away. This…this sensation…was searing; it hurt. It was acute, bulging, bursting, penetrating, the urge to bear down, and that was merely the physical. Mentally, it was the challenge of sustaining the pain, giving in to the pain, coping with the pain—an entirely different kind of pain, the kind of pain that literally makes one moo-howl-roar.

It was the unknown. How much longer? How much more of this can I stand? Indeed, the reaction is not only to pull away, but to run, hightail it.

Even so, this cow-wolf-bear, she was hearty. And the ol' nag was her biggest cheerleader…or button-pusher.

Don't you dare! There is no way out! This is what you wanted! the ol' windbag badgered as my knees tamped the mattress below.

Shut up, you ol' heifer. I blew her off and blew through pursed lips, attempting to pull myself together, wondering why I wasn't handling this differently. Better. Whatever that entailed. Less animalistic, maybe. Before I lunged at the wall, that sound escaping me a second time, convinced I could either go through it or up it.

That's the big fat *cow* calling the kettle black! The *heifer* antagonized, in her own twisted way supporting the *moo*-howl-roar.

So I tamped the wall, the magnified whites of my eyes looking, searching, assessing, as if I might actually find danger. To my right was Wade. To my left was Genevieve. I must have looked wild and scared. I did not want to be wild and scared. Damn reality! Why can't you just let me have my fantasy? I am supposed to be loving and laughing and reminiscing, birthing this child into serenity. *Serenity Now!*

Did I want to whisper, plead, "Help me." Or did I want to shout, demand, "HELP ME!"

They are helping you, ya big boob! You wanted to get primal! Old, reptilian, lizard, yada blah yada, something brain, remember! Why did you go to the trouble of crafting a Chant Sheet if you aren't even gonna use the damn thing!

Chant Sheet? Yes, the ol' scalawag was right! Chant Sheet, page two, fifth paragraph down: "If you are to give birth instinctively, spontaneously, drug-free, there is virtually nowhere to go but *through* your pain."

Through my pain, through my pain, through my pain, I chanted. But can't I go through it differently? Serenely? Calmly? Breezily? Oh, sweet Jesus, here comes more of that pain. Pain I tried to outmaneuver, pull away from, before another unbecoming moo-howl-roar discharged itself from my bowels.

Good God, what is that sound? And why do I keep making it!

Give it up, princess! You ain't birthin' peacefully!

But listen to me! I must be scaring Mila. I *am* my mother's pet peeve—"a screamer"—or worse, a moo-howl-roarer. What is Wade going to think? I am probably scaring him, too, turning him off for a lifetime! Genevieve is probably wondering what she got herself into, taking the moo-howl-roarer on as a client.

You think she hasn't heard it all! Are you that self-absorbed! That concerned with your social self!

No! I just want everyone to be comfortable. *I* want to be comfortable. Listen to me! I contested, as there liberated another moo-howl-roar. I must be scaring the whole neighborhood.

*Listen* to yourself! Get out of your head and into your body! Mind, ego, inhibitions, to the background! The ol' nag started paraphrasing the Chant Sheet, or Shout Sheet, rather. Forget everything you think you know! Just let it happen! Trust! Surrender! Accept! Your body knows how to do this, dammit!

Moo (Yes)! Howl (It)! Roar (Does)!

# Adventure Of A Lifetime

"THE WAY A SOCIETY VIEWS A PREGNANT AND BIRTHING WOMAN REFLECTS HOW that society views women as a whole. If women are considered weak in their most powerful moments, what does that mean?" —Marcie Macari

Genevieve and Katie were joined by Erica, partnering midwife who attends from transition on to ensure adequate hands on deck. These three women in the room with me, in the thick of my birth, did not consider me weak even though I moo-howl-roared like a wounded cow-wolf-bear.

These women knew something I did not.

Transition, in any process and explicitly in birth, can be intimidating, exhausting, seemingly impossible.

These women knew that I was experiencing the quintessential transition.

I now understand all the attention allocated to transition labor and coping: "How to Get Through Transition Without an Epidural," "6 Tips On What To Do In Transition Labor," "Transition: The Most Intense Stage of Labor."

Even pro-transition attention: "Why I Love Transition Labor (And You Might Too)."[1]

What?!

"I have to say, had I been in the hospital...," I talked to Genevieve, Katie, and Erica moments after our home birth, reliving the intensity of it all, "...with that whole transition bit, I would have wanted the epidural."

"Anyone would have," they assuaged my admission.

Feeling jovial with a safe and successful home birth in the books, my epidural comment—be it laced in gleeful gratitude and delivered en passant the way an insurance company may address fine print—was no laughing matter.

I meant what I said: I would have wanted the epidural.

Would I have taken it? I will never know. Nonexistent in my home birth, I thought no more about an epidural than I did a cesarean. Did I need it? Was it essential? No.

And that sums up transition, in general, and in birth specifically. Doing/going through something that may be the hardest thing ever… and doing it anyway. Understanding that the essentials reside within us. There are no quick fixes. We may have to sit in it for a spell. Change is coming with or without us. We may as well accept it. See where it takes us. Might the accomplishment outweigh the work—the effort, the uncertainty, the pain.

But you know none of this during transition.

I have read about some women who thought they might actually die while giving life, in transition labor. It is that hard. It is that much of a mindfuck. Sorry, Ma, I know of no other term as nail-on-the-head accurate.

I never felt as though I was going to die, but I did wonder if I might just pass out. It felt a realistic possibility from the shock and stress of it all.

Yes, "shock" and "stress," two words that are synonymous with "trauma."

There can be trauma in childbirth, physical and emotional. Depending on women's birthing experiences, from caregiver to intervention to outcome, there can be birth battle scars. I have read birth stories as intense and captivating as war stories. And I am convinced that if men gave birth, birth stories would be told more like war stories, chock-full of challenge, hardship, suspense, and valor! There are women who suffer from post-traumatic stress disorder, distinct from postpartum depression, in direct relationship to their birthing experience.

That said, my hospital birth with no transition at all was closer to my personal definition of "traumatic" than I ever thought of my home birth transition being. Although my home birth transition *was* challenging enough, stressful enough, shocking enough that what I can recollect is piddly compared to what I cannot.

I jokingly, yet not so jokingly, refer to this lost time as "transition amnesia." I empathize with Goldie Hawn's "Annie" in the 1987 romantic comedy *Overboard*, who suffered from true and clinical amnesia: "Ever since I walked through that door I've done nothing but cook, clean, scrub, chop wood. I've looked after you, your dogs, your kids and your friends so that I might remember one shred of my life here and now it's clear to me why I have chosen to block it out!"

Leading me to wonder is "transition amnesia" like pain in labor? Is it purposeful? Some protective old brain/knowing body connection that provides amnesic pain relief? The body—too stressed, shocked, utterly taxed with its current job—requires the brain to play catch-up in an attempt to cope, where the brain is then too busy coping to even store the memory?

That place between Laborland and Birthland—Transition—was murky, similar to early labor but deprived of the dreaminess. What I remember of it seemed maybe fifteen minutes. Wade said it was much longer. It had to be. Right?

I remember Genevieve breaking my bag of waters and how great that felt. I remember the first few moo-howl-roars and arguing with the ol' nag and being completely naked—without a tinker's damn—on all fours in the middle of my bed like some cow-wolf-bear and thinking I would not get through it. How could I? I remember feeling strangely out of sorts, confused by the contractions, the sensations. Did I have to puke? Poop? Push? Pass out? Explode? Implode? They all seemed viable, imminent, possibly simultaneous! I remember the ol' nag winning, my body winning, apparently and finally my mind disappearing into it and pressing onward.

Then the next thing I recall is squatting on the birthing stool, where Genevieve was massaging away a cervical lip on an otherwise fully dilated me. But I have no recollection of how I got there, when I got there—the transition from transitioning to pushing.

"Labor works best when you're out of your mind," said a quote from my Chant Sheet.

No doubt, it did.

And if I had not prepared to *lose my marbles*, I easily could have. The pain, the confusion, the fear, it would have been effortless to let panic conquer. To flee, to leave my body, to creep back into my mind, begging consciousness and logic for a "fix" they could not deliver.

I read about this in my preparation, women corroborating that transition was the turning point where the mind and the body may un-sync, attempting to turn against one another. Keep going, they said. Don't give in to fear, they said. Generations of women have done it, so can you, they said. Your baby waits…just on the other side of this transition, they said. Dig in, push through, stay with her, go to him, meet them there, it will be glorious, they said.

Pain is temporary. Fear is about the future. Do not be afraid. Be in the moment. One contraction. One rest. One push. One of anything is nothing more than you can handle. Be curious. Be open. Go to the edge and beyond, my Chant Sheet said, subconsciously.

The external inspiration as encouraging, Genevieve empowered without many words at all. She empowered with patience and presence—relaxed of breath and face, almost a gentle smile, modestly attending. There was no commotion, no big to-do. No people coming and going, busily preparing, although she and Katie and Erica did prepare respectfully, without interference or announcement. Self-limiting background players, it was not their birth, their delivery; it was ours. One step ahead of us the entire time—absorbent underpads here and there, birthing stool, position changes, handheld Doppler, direction, anything and everything—we lacked nothing.

Most importantly, the belief in me, my body, the process…was there.

I did not need rescuing.

Transition surprised me. That's all. What I needed was *time…* enough to adjust to the intensity. Enough to wrap my mind around transition and recommit my body to it. Enough to trust, to surrender, to accept that transition was the new, and temporary, normal.

The women in the room, they knew this, too. They knew that once we made it through the tunnel of Transition, the light on the other side would carry and literally push us on to Birthland.

They knew what author Sheryl Feldman knew when she wrote, "There is power that comes to women when they give birth. They don't ask for it, it simply invades them. Accumulates like clouds on the horizon and passes through, carrying the child with it."

Even Wade, my home birth skeptic, did not treat me as though I needed rescuing. If ever there was a time I felt I might, transition was that time. But he felt it, too. The edge, the electricity, something waited for us…in the air, in the room, in the space.

"Felt it?" he piped. "Hell, I *heard* it! That noise you were making. 'Grrrhhh!'"

Power.

It must leach out of birthing bones, cavernous, untapped—untested. Capable yet submissive, it weathers contraction after contraction where there is no leverage, no control, only the faculty to try and try again.

Power.

I used to think it was in a muscle, how much that muscle could lift, how much that muscle could endure. I used to think it was in a voice, how far that voice could project, the range that voice could manipulate. I used to think it was explosion, a sprint, a jab, how fast legs and arms could go from zero to sixty. Will, yes, power was will—"willpower"—determination to get something done. *Do* something.

Power is in stillness. Power is in knowing it is coming back…again and again…yet squatting in it, *doing* nothing. Feet to the floor and holding the line, no retreat but total surrender.

Power is stillness? Power is surrender?

I never would have believed it, comprehended it, without experiencing it.

It was me. I was there. On that birthing stool, after transition and fully dilated and preparing to push. But it was no me that I had ever encountered before. That woman and that man—my birth warrior and Wade's birth coach warrior—were never so powerful as in the surrender of transition and in the stillness directly thereafter.

On the precipice of something greater than we had ever endured/

achieved/come through individually or as a couple, discovering our limits went far beyond any boundary we could have imagined.

A trial of physical and mental and spiritual wherewithal, birth is as challenging to the mind and body as it is rewarding to the soul. There *will* be times you feel you have nothing left. The end *will* come. Comprised of equal parts elation and exhaustion, that end will carry with it immense pride and relief. All to be outweighed by an overwhelming humility and reverence for the wonder and magnitude of *life*.

For you have just given it. Surrendered to it. Let it come through you. Born it into the world. *Life*.

Talk about the adventure of a *life*time. And we didn't even have to leave home.

# Look What She Just Did

I HAD READ AND HEARD IT SAID THAT PUSHING IS A *RELIEF*: A FEELING OF reassurance and ~~relaxation~~ following release from anxiety or distress.

Nix "relaxation" and, yes, relief is a suitable definition for the pushing phase.

"Reassurance" being the operative word, pushing provided encouragement. Pushing provided direction. Like a switch, everything that was confusing and confidence-crushing in transition was instantly clear and certain. The finish line manifesting, it felt to me a second wind, if you are a runner...or a child at bedtime.

I wondered would I fancy "laboring down"? Labor down, breathe, rest, maintain and be thankful, allowing baby to drop lower into the pelvis before bearing down.

I wanted to fancy laboring down. Yes, another fantasy.

"Oh, you're gonna push," Wade had said, his brows upraising, as if to add, *if you think you aren't pushing, you got another think coming!*

Little shit.

I pushed.

It matched my personality. It was rewarding and relieving, likely and exactly what I needed to do in that moment, in that birth.

Chalk it up to positioning, but once I got on the birthing stool, the urge to push seemed inescapable.

I did have a bit of an anterior lip, which basically means I was fully dilated but the anterior edge of my cervix was a tad swollen and still in the way of baby's head. The management of the cervical lip can be somewhat controversial. Some providers believe it is best to avoid pushing until the cervical lip has disappeared whether by natural or mechanical forces, regardless of a woman's urge. Other providers view the cervical lip as a normal physiological process, and that a birthing woman should push through it if compelled to do so. That attempting to prevent spontaneous pushing—unstoppable and undirected pushing—at this stage could lead to more rather than less problems.

I had read, and was of a mind to believe, that a cervical lip *was* normal. It made sense to me that most women—at some point in labor, whether identified or not—will have an anterior cervical lip because anatomically it is the last part of the cervix to be pulled up over baby's head.

Genevieve's and my effort was a collaboration. She did not dissuade me from pushing, but rather worked with my urge to do so in diminishing my cervical lip. It took next to nothing in terms of time, maybe two pushes and a few massaging maneuvers. I could neither tell nor feel what she did exactly, too preoccupied with feeling the imminent and impulsive and afflictive sensation of pushing.

In the meantime, Wade and I tried out a few birth partner support positions conducive to the birthing stool before finding one that fit. I couldn't even do that the way I might have envisioned, appreciating and encouraging him with something such as "You've been the best birth partner. I couldn't have done it without you. We're almost there. Baby's almost here. I love you."

Flower-child birther I am never going to be, Xena moo-howl-roared, "You're pulling me back. Don't do it like that. I gotta be up like this. You're pulling me back!"

*Tougher Than the Rest*, Wade did not roar back or hold it against me while he held himself against me in support squat position.

I had also read and heard it said, "Push like you're having the biggest bowel movement of your life."

Okay…

Pushing felt quite natural. I could wrap my abs and core around the push, inherently knowing how to maneuver with the contraction. "How" savvied. Wrapping my mind around the "where" was a bit foreign. Where do I direct the ejection? Out? Down? Somewhere other than in?

Genevieve knew exactly how to help with that, too. Purposely avoiding the directive "push," she recognized my body's natural birth physiology, its "urge" to bear down.

"Here," she said, "when you feel that urge, direct it here," her finger gently pressing against what felt to me the back of my vagina. More specifically, the distal exterior wall of my vagina that runs parallel to the rectum behind it…à la "the biggest bowel movement of your life."

That tidbit provided noteworthy guidance, the difference in pushing to push and pushing with purpose, which only heartened my confidence. Yes, I *can* do this. I know *how* and *where* to do this.

In several different positions for pushing, supported squat on the birthing stool kicked things off. In no particular order thereafter, I recall hands and knees, forward-leaning, semi-sitting, side-lying, and flat on my back. That one surprised me. I was not expecting it. I had not envisioned it.

I had focused so deeply on avoiding the mistakes I made in my hospital birth, where I spent far too much time on my back and in bed, anything remotely close would seem counterintuitive. Lying on my back for a series of pushes facilitated passing baby's head below my pubic bone, otherwise known as internal rotation.

Each position, encouraged by Genevieve, was intended to foster baby and me through the "seven cardinal movements"—engagement, descent, flexion, internal rotation, extension, external rotation, expulsion.

My focus on enduring, getting baby out, and getting over all of the acutely agonizing sensations that make up the pushing phase, I wish I would have had the wherewithal to direct my focus to each of the cardinal movements. To cling to them, to capture and hold on to those last moments of birth, rather short-lived compared to an overall lingering labor. But I found it hard to appreciate much beyond the finish line, the hunt for relief.

Unable to identify the cardinal movements individually, I could feel a difference overall as baby passed through me. Sensations distinct yet compounding, there was a crescendo to crowning: From a crushing-cramping, Oh, Lord, I have to poop! To a twisting-wringing and widening-expanding, Good God, how much more can my bones and ligaments stand! To an abrupt pulling-stretching—some say "ring of fire"—and pulsing-burning-thrilling-tingling, Oh, sweet Jesus, hair! I can feel hair!

Not only aiding the literal passage of a child, the continual change in position aided in making bearable the grueling rite of passage. Just as I would start to think I can't possibly push anymore, Genevieve would suggest a new position, which for whatever reason made it easier to continue pushing. Momentum, would be my guess. Each reposition championed momentum, forward progress.

It was this momentum—doing, managing, endgame—part of labor that felt expeditious. It seemed maybe thirty minutes, if that. Wade said it was much longer. It had to be. Right?

One thing is certain, it was the part of labor in which I felt I thrived. Easily? Magically? Effortlessly? Nope! Moo-howl-roaring the entire way, and actually audibly praying for the first time in my labor, when I imagined I would pray more.

On all fours in the middle of our bed between pushing with contractions, and with my head bowed to my pillow, I vividly recall praying, "Lord, please give me the strength."

And Genevieve said, "Amen."

I loved that she said this. It helped in a way. Regardless of her beliefs, she validated mine. What a lovely confirmation in my birth. I will never forget how she whispered "amen" when I needed Him to hear me, anyone to hear me.

It seems as though I pushed through about five contractions per position, my spontaneous pushing rhythm maybe five to ten seconds per push and maybe three to five pushes total per contraction. The time between contractions seemed nonexistent at this point, basically enough to catch a breath, maybe reposition, and press on. The longest duration between contractions had to be the last few contractions, after baby's head was born and we were waiting for another and another to push the body through. Everything decelerated then, or at least felt as though it did, *Chariots of Fire* slow-motion on the homestretch.

If only I could recall in what reference I first read about the notion of a woman feeling with her own hand the movement of her child down into the vagina, and at crowning, as a guide to how much work was left and how hard or not to push. Whichever book it was, I found the idea riveting. Definitely something I wanted to do, not only for the direction I was certain it provided but for the feeling, the memory, the first touch of our child. And to do that while our child was still within my body? How extraordinary. What an inspiration that must be to push through to meeting baby.

I hoped it would be innate, specifically after becoming aware of it. But I had a sneaking suspicion that it might not resonate in a one-track-get-this-baby-out mind. So I broached the subject with Genevieve and let it be known that when it comes to physical modesty I am no *Girls Gone Wild*, but I am Girl Gone Renaissance—eager to know and experience.

"If I don't remember to feel for baby, by all means, please take my hand and remind me," I said.

And she did, at a pivotal moment, no less. On the birthing stool—not the first time but for another position change—I distinctly remember how open I felt and how easily palpable baby's head was. Soft and speckled with hair, the evocative memory still gives me goose-bumps. The inspiration, confirmation, and renewed dedication that one direction provided cannot be overlooked. We had been pushing for what felt a fairly substantial stretch, and I could not help but wonder if it was working at all.

"Feel that? That's baby's head," Genevieve coached with a smile.

"Yeah," I whisper-panted, smiling back.

Feeling that soft round itty-bitty noggin scantly flecked with hair and bravely emerging, embracing the challenge, the embodiment of new life...gave new life to the pushing. Not quite a finger length, and I have relatively long fingers, we had a ways to go. But feeling gave me a point of reference, improved visualization. Totally doable, it never felt closer.

By the time baby was crowning, it *had* become innate. My hand seemingly attached to my labia, I felt the progression from a piggy bank slot to an open chatterbox—origami fortune teller—the progression from a spot of hair on the crown of a head palpable with a fingertip to a widow's peak silhouetted with hair on a grapefruit-sized head filling an entire palm.

The grapefruit image was only fitting and helpful, another Chant Sheet paraphrase from a birthing woman in another Ina May Gaskin book: "I'm going to get huge. Grapefruit, huge. Big. Not just ten centimeters big, bigger than the baby. I'm going to get huge."

And I did.

Shut my mouth wide open!

I was there. I felt it. I did it. Well, technically, my vagina did it. Yet it still amazes me.

Sure, the uterus is amazing. Accepting of implantation, placental attachment and growth, production of the perfect sterile environment, encapsulating and incubating a baby, I think we can all agree that the uterus is truly stunning.

But the vagina…she ain't too shabby.

Frankly, I was too impressed with her to worry would she ever be the same. More mature? Worse for wear? A little tear?

Look what she just did!

She dazzled Wade, too. "I still can't believe you pushed our son out of your vagina. I wasn't sure how I'd feel about that," he paused. "But it was so…'grrrhhh!'" There he went growling, mocking my moo-howl-roar again. "Sexy, babe. Is that weird? I want you more than ever."

No, it is not weird. It's sweet. Exactly what a weeks' postpartum wife wants to hear. I imagine it is only natural considering what we came through together. Like few other one-of-a-kind undertakings—the physical and emotional and spiritual test of it all—the result of trial and triumph was a stronger bond.

# Pushy

Now then, rewind a few months and that same *sweet* husband of mine made not the slightest attempt at honeying his words when he said, "You might as well plan on tearing, babe. Your personality, you're just gonna blow right through it."

"How can you avoid pushing...," he continued before pausing, maybe considering the risk of offending me, "...when you're pushy."

"Pushy?" I said, offended, but guilty.

"Yes, ba-a-abe...pushy."

"Yet you're here, we're here, about to have kid number two."

"I didn't say I didn't like it. I love that about you."

That I'm pushy? I internalized the thought.

"That you're a go-getter, hell yes, that's attractive," he replied, reading my mind.

To which I internalized some more, oh, don't go changing the tone now that you've already called me pushy. I know I push myself, but..."Do I push you?"

"No, yes, sometimes."

"I do?"

"You can't help yourself, babe, it's in your blood."

Oh, but, one *can* help herself. I choked back that thought, too, even though I meant it.

"Sometimes I need a push. We're a good team that way, you push, I pull." He did it again, read my mind and eased it, smiling all sexy and understanding, moving in on me and the bump, hands and arms *pulling* us to him. "You do you and I'll do me...maybe I can pull you back from pushing so much in labor."

Tell that to the laboring couple who waited nearly a year to lay eyes on their child. Tell that to the laboring couple who previously miscarried, uncertain they would ever lay eyes on new life constructed of their DNA. Tell that to the laboring couple who labored all day and who are finally a few good pushes away from laying eyes on the child they waited nearly a year to see.

Tell that to the laboring woman whose body has been bearing the brunt of labor all day and who knows the only way to stop the force is to "get this baby out!"

I did tear, a smidge.

*But*, I didn't "blow right through it." See, ba-a-abe, "Pushy" *can* refrain.

Anyone who has ever participated in a birthing class with other expectant moms and dads knows that the topic of tearing needs no introduction. Concerns about tearing and how to prevent it are usually right up there with concerns about pain and how to cope with it, possibly taking up an entire class itself.

Tearing seems so intimidating because it is so indeterminate. Impossible to predict or prevent, who tears exactly and why is unknown, in the least unclear.

There is a greater likelihood of tearing in first-time vaginal deliveries, yet it can happen in subsequent vaginal deliveries all the same. Positioning has much to do with the probability of tearing, but what position? Some believe squatting opens everything wider and aids in not tearing, while others believe squatting predisposes tearing because of the pressure it puts on the perineum. Birthing a baby in OP/"sunny-side up" position can increase the risk of tearing, yet birthing a baby in OA/"optimal" position can and does result in tearing as well. Demographics influence tearing, with Asian women specifically at risk because their babies have on average larger head circumference per the standard growth chart, yet there are babies of various ethnic backgrounds with substantial noggins and women of various ethnic backgrounds who experience tears.

Perineal massage, perineal counter pressure, perineal warm compress—are any of these modalities efficacious in preventing tearing? Does pushing cause tearing? Are birthing women pushing too hard, too soon?

A question that has earned its own descriptor, the "push paradox," supposes that when it comes to pushing in labor, "more isn't better." Arguably applicable to rearing children and birthing them—whether trying to get them to participate in the class play or trying to get them out of your vagina—pushiness may not be the best approach.

Ina May Gaskin wrote of multiparous women—having one or more previous births—that Amish women specifically, whom she witnessed, birth "effortlessly." These women had learned to allow the uterus to do the work while they maintained their focus on relaxation in their bodies and through contractions. Such relaxation and "laboring down" provide the uterus the groundwork for swift birthing.

What a way to birth *and* stay intact, I thought. Although I was unable to adhere to the notion in my own and first vaginal birth...feeling the desire, the need, the urge to push.

Why does tearing have to be so perplexing? How is it that we have yet to ascertain a way to avoid it unequivocally? Is it just one of those things, like cesarean, that "happens" to some of us but not to others?

One thing I am certain of is this: I can thank my midwife that I only tore a smidge. There was no intervention, no induction, no epidural, no forceps, no vacuum, no directed *Push! Push! Push!* All of which have been proven to increase the risk and severity of perineal damage.

Taking into account my pushy personality, I am also certain that I could have done my perineum a favor in laboring down, in relaxing, in holding back in pushing the pushing along. As Ina May depicted, I could have waited for it to come to me and allowed my uterus to do the work.

In addition, I have to think that asymptomatic and possible preexisting pelvic floor impairment from years of running, and other high-impact activities, did my perineum no favors in the tearing department. I say "possible preexisting" because symptoms did not manifest until my postpartum healing.

Couple all of that with suboptimal diet and body mechanics, as I am convinced we neither eat nor move the way anthropology may have us believe we were biologically and physiologically designed to, and I should probably be praising my perineum for only tearing a smidge.

I have found no scientific evidence/method to prove this belief. Where would we find such statistics of our primary ancestors' predisposition to vaginal tearing? Absurd, right. But thought-provoking, nonetheless.

What was childbirth like for the "cavewoman" who mastered Body Mechanics 101 in infancy with the basic flat-footed resting squat and never had the modern comforts of the chair, couch, seat, stool? One can watch a toddler at play and recognize the innate ability and proper body mechanics to squat. Now imagine that squat—naturally lengthening *and* strengthening muscles, ligaments, core, glutes, pelvic floor, perineum—is the norm, the natural state of relaxation, and how that would bode well for any birthing woman.

Ina May Gaskin said, "Squat 300 times a day, you're going to give birth quickly."

It is too controversial, and arguably unprovable, to pinpoint what the cavewoman ate. However, if we knew exactly—some postulate her weight in nutrient-rich and diverse wild greens from naturally robust soil, as well as *the whole beast*—and had the *guts* to eat it, too, might our diets better support the perineum and surrounding tissues in labor? For essential vitamins and minerals and proteins, often lacking in a modern diet, perform the most basic work in all bodily cells, supporting the balance, function, and structure of all bodily organs and tissues, right down to the perineum.

Try as I may, I do not eat to the cavewoman's standard. Do I want to squat 300 times a day? Probably couldn't if I tried! But I am working on it, and it is improving my pelvic floor.

I did, nevertheless, squat over a mirror at the six-week mark taking my first postpartum peek.

My heart went lub-dub, lub-dub, lub-dub, squatting over that mirror in the solitude of my bathroom. I had prepared for this. Birth, vaginal birth, has to change the landscape "down there." Why was I so nervous? Other than the possibility I would not recognize my own vagina!

Only to ultimately wonder was I more relieved or disappointed when there she was identifiable and unremarkable, no trace of a battle scar, no distinguishing "I gave birth" characteristics.

"Hmm…," I exhaled, putting away the mirror.

"Everything okay?" Wade asked upon my bathroom exit, lurking, as curious as I.

"Looks like she always has," I said, mid shrug.

"Well, that's good, right?"

"You tell me."

"What'd you expect?"

"I don't know." I shrugged again. "I guess I thought she might look a little more…dignified?" I couldn't help but join Wade in snickering at my choice of adjective.

"I've heard a fair share of words describing vaginas, babe, and 'dignified' ain't one of 'em." He took a long pause before repeating, "Dignified?"

"Yeah, you know, it might look like it favors…tea and crumpets and…talks with a British accent," I defended through a red-faced smile at my ridiculous self. "I mean, she *should* be knighted or something."

"They don't knight women, babe." Was he seriously getting into specifics about my hypothetical dignified British vagina? "She'd be a lady. No, maybe a dame…"

"Ooh, da-a-a-me," I interrupted, "I like that. Dame…'Pushy.'" *Obviously* I had let it go that he thought me pushy.

He gave me a discerning squint before mediating with wit and a horribly amusing British accent. "Well, then, doth Dame 'Pushy' care to be squired by Lord Lure?" The fisherman in him was much too proud of his counter-title ripe with innuendo.

How I cackled, at his shtick *and* at the thought of sex, a sincere offer camouflaged in the cheekiness of his jest.

Whilst I was assured by this point that vaginas, birthing vaginas, my vagina was in fact supernatural, capable not only of defying the laws of nature but of pretty much anything, the first postpartum lovemaking would have to wait. Having much in common with the first postpartum bowel movement, the psychological was harder to overcome than the actual.

It would take more time for me to discover that it was nothing a lay cook's recipe could not cure—glass of wine, dash of courage, pinch of patience, dollop of coconut oil, and enjoy!

# The Body That Birth Built

A DEAR AND DELECTABLE FRIEND WHO HANGS OUT IN MY HEART MORE THAN with me these days—I with toddlers and she with teenagers—told me in my first pregnancy, "Nothing is ever going to be the same. Your life, your priorities, your sleep, your body...*nothing is ever going to be the same.*"

I was willing to accept that, with one naive exception. A bit big for my britches, I actually thought I could circumvent the metamorphoses that pregnancy and birth and breastfeeding bring on a body. With heartfelt humility, I now concede to the fact that there are changes a pregnant and birthing and nursing body go through that no amount of strength training and conditioning or good nutrition can restore.

Oddly enough, the one thing that even the pre-pregnancy me was certain *would* change post-pregnancy, and post-vaginal birth specifically, is the only thing that remains unchanged!

Do not let me mislead. It was not painless. My perineum was swollen and inflamed and implored of me to move, and sit, most gingerly for the first week. I eagerly and attentively partook in homeopathic applications, such as perineal washes and perineal ice packs infused with Happy Mama Herbals postpartum sitz bath, around the clock for the first week while relieving pain and healing perineal tissue.

For the first few days, not only my perineum but every muscle on my body ached, as though I had endured the toughest workout of my life. Patchy and tiny purple splotches bedecked my face, chest, and arms from broken blood vessels. My upper lip—apparently pressed and stretched across my teeth as I moo-howl-roared—was so swollen that it looked like a lip-injection caricature. I assume these were signs that I did push too aggressively. Then again, maybe every woman has such, or different, push-aches and birth battle scars.

By the end of the second week, I was quite comfortable. Another four weeks out, at the quintessential six-week mark, I was back to full activity, even able to partake in running and strength training again.

Anyone who has birthed vaginally may not be surprised in the least. But I was. Although I pushed a wee human out of my vagina and snagged her a bit in the process, recovery was effortless compared to that required after my cesarean.

Just enough postpartum normalcy before ushering in another revelation.

Labor, I prepared for that. Pain, I prepared for that. Birth, I prepared for that. Patiently healing, I prepared for that. Tearing, though convinced I would not, I was even prepared for that.

Leaking when I sneeze? Who prepares for that!

When lochia—normal postpartum bleeding/discharge—stopped and I got off the potty, done and wiped, I felt a little dribble. My first thought was, ah, excuse me, what was that? I lied to myself the first few times, oh, it must be a little more lochia. When it kept happening, I knew better.

So I started keeping track. It did not happen every time, but intermittently enough to cause concern. And here I thought everything was great, back to a hundred percent.

I confided in Genevieve. She always has pointers and brought to my attention the new studies on squatting and how it relates to pelvic floor health versus the previously recommended Kegel.[1] She also directed me to the "client information packet" I received from her upon my first prenatal visit with a section on "post-pregnancy core rebuilding," which aids in pelvic floor support. Notably, the core rebuilding exercises were devoid of the ubiquitous sit-up, which increases unfavorable intra-abdominal/downward pressure on the pelvic organs and supporting structures.

Katie, Genevieve's apprentice, shared with me a fascinating and very affordable toilet trinket called the "Squatty Potty." The Squatty Potty recreates a squatting experience of sorts more comparable to the way we were designed to relieve ourselves. This made great sense, as I had shared with them that squatting over the potty instead of sitting on it eliminated the dribble, which I discovered only after using a public toilet, of course.

They both encouraged me to give my body time. "Be kind to your body." "Be patient with yourself." "Take time to heal." I can still recall Genevieve's gentle guidance after our miscarriage.

Armed with new information, I went away inspired to learn more.

First things first, what precisely is a "pelvic floor"? And why is mine malfunctioning?

The pelvic floor is the area beneath the pelvic cavity and above the perineum. Composed of muscle and connective tissue, one can think of the pelvic floor as a girdle or a hammock with a bit of a trampoline-like quality that supports pelvic organs—bladder, uterus, vagina, small bowel, and rectum—and also contributes to their function.

It is said, and reasonable to see, that pregnancy and childbirth can "weaken" the pelvic floor, given the strain that both pose on pelvic organs and their supporting structures.

However, I was unconvinced that I did not have some form of pelvic floor dysfunction, even if mild and asymptomatic, prior to pregnancy and birth.

I did not encounter any symptomatic pelvic floor issues in my first prenatal or postpartum experience. One could chalk it up to cesarean birth? Although, I have read and heard that some women who birth via cesarean do have pelvic floor issues, whether arising from pregnancy or partial labor or potentially long labor prior to cesarean or some other reason outside of pregnancy. In fact, women, and men, who have never been pregnant can and do experience pelvic floor hurdles.

Without a prior vaginal birth, I had nothing to compare the cesarean aspect. Yet I did have a partial and what I would consider lengthy labor prior to my cesarean. In hindsight, it is very clear to me that my pregnancies were night and day in the pelvic floor department. It remains a bit of an enigma that my first carried so easily but carried in the least optimal birthing position, while my last did not carry easily at all but carried in the most optimal birthing position. Even though they both technically weighed the same at birth, I think back on how heavily my last carried. Not only in my uterus but in my bones and muscles and connective tissues and on my bladder, unexpectedly causing me to give up running by the middle of the second trimester due to the sheer discomfort of it.

Was that my pelvic floor forewarning? Hey, you, I could use a little TLC here!

With each consecutive pregnancy and birth does the pelvic floor take more of a beating? Was it the combination of pregnancy and birthing and age and even a first-degree perineal tear? One month shy of forty in my last birth, I was experiencing them simultaneously. Or was my pelvic floor simply not in the best shape to begin with?

Imagine my wake-up call in learning that running during pregnancy, and in general, can lead to pelvic floor "give way," as the impact and jarring of the running stride and motion is not particularly kind to the trampoline-like sling of the pelvic floor. My first ribbon earned at five years of age for being the youngest to complete a 5K, which I accompanied my older sister, I have been a runner all my life.

Urinary incontinence is problematic for female Olympians, with runners and gymnasts having the highest percentage. Yes, urinary incontinence is relatively frequent among young *childless* elite athletes who partake in high-impact sports that demand maximum effort. What? Beyond fit, at the pinnacle of strength and conditioning, how can *they* have pelvic floor dysfunction?

It is the intensity, the excessive intra-abdominal pressure repetitively overloading pelvic organs, forcing them downwards and injuring supporting structures. Intense repetitive motion is no friend to the pelvic floor. Dancers, performing ballet specifically, and even simply "physically active" women are prone to "stress incontinence," one study reporting forty-seven percent of them experience it after vaginal deliveries.[2]

Hands down, the most surprising element post-vaginal birth for this "physically active" woman was the pelvic floor issue. In retrospect, I could not help but think "tearing schmearing," talk to me about pelvic floor. Surely an entire birthing class could be allocated to pelvic floor health, a topic that may not figuratively weigh as heavily as tearing but literally does.

Initially, it was confusing. Is this what happens? Is this my new post-partum norm? It's underreported to begin with. Some who are bold enough to talk about it have the attitude that "it is what it is." And *it* is. Just ask Poise, TENA, Prevail, and tens of other incontinence hygiene providers.

But what if there is something I can do about it or at least help correct the underlying condition? To which I stumbled upon "Why Postpartum Urinary Incontinence is NOT Normal (and How to Fix It)" and "Leaking When You Laugh Is NOT Normal—The Truth About Postpartum Urinary Incontinence."

Equally confounding is the fact that some countries are ahead of the curve in "postpartum pelvic floor health," where they promote awareness and education and referral to "women's health physiother-apists" whose primary specialty is arming postpartum women with noninvasive and practical information to restore function of the pelvic floor. Why are we not one of those countries? Several Australia and New Zealand studies highlight the efficacy of physiotherapy in "pelvic floor muscle training," further highlighting that improvements at six months after physiotherapy were the same as those after pelvic floor surgery, where physiotherapy is six percent the cost of surgery.[3]

Whilst I did not go to a physiotherapist, I personally and habitually rehabilitated my pelvic floor. I figured it was similar to piano lessons: it was not who taught the lesson that mattered so much as the practice, the application.

It took its fair share of time and retraining. But I could tell an im-mediate difference after studying and improving my overall squat form and including squatting in daily activity versus exclusively in work-outs—maybe like the "cavewoman" we talked about previously.

A lover of strength training, I was familiar with squats and enjoyed them occasionally as part of my regimen. Albeit, as author and bio-mechanist Katy Bowman's runaway blog post pointed out, "You (Still) Don't Know Squat."[4]

It turns out the intermittent squatting I did inherently in my pregnancy for the relief it provided is more than just relieving. It is ingrained in our most basic physiology. "Squatting is essentially a position of the body that humans have used for thousands of years, and in many cultures is still being used today."[5]

We are built to squat. From an evolutionary or anatomical or anthropological perspective, we are fundamentally built for deep flat-footed resting squats. Not just at the gym but at home, at the park, at the grocery store, at work, and at play. Consciously capitalizing on the squat, I employ it in any instance where I might otherwise bend over. I squat at the grocery store to choose items from the bottom shelf. I squat alongside my squatting children in playing with them. I squat while loading and unloading the dishwasher, while pulling and folding clothes from the dryer, intermittently throughout the day as and where I am of a mind to. Not for any particular length of time, a few seconds here, a few minutes there. And it is paying off, particularly in the pelvic floor health department.

In my understanding and personal experience, there is not one thing better equipped at *strengthening* while concurrently *lengthening* than a deep flat-footed resting squat—the natural range of motion of a natural human being. This *strength-length* relationship is the key component to a healthy pelvic floor.

The pelvic floor must be *long* enough not to be hypertonic/short, which results in increased pressure and abnormal tone that can manifest in pelvic, groin, and lower back pain, as well as difficulty in urination and defecation and/or "urge incontinence"—inability to hold back urine long enough to get to a bathroom. The pelvic floor must be *strong* enough not to be hypotonic/weak, which results in a lax tone that can manifest in organ prolapse and/or "stress incontinence"—leakage of urine with any increased abdominal pressure such as laughing, coughing, sneezing or exercising.

Basically, the strength-length relationship of the pelvic floor is required to support the function of one's body and pelvic organs throughout daily activities, as well as provide extra bursts of support coinciding with intermittent and instantaneous increases in abdominal pressure. This basic function of the pelvic floor is pivotal in pointing out the importance of mental retraining, too, in thinking about posture and core stability and how one carries herself.

Naturally a bit disturbing at first, the postpartum dribble only enriched my body mechanics. I have enjoyed the lesson. With conscious and habitual engagement of my core while sitting or standing or squatting and with attention to my pelvic floor—proper movements done in proper form that facilitate function—I am now able to cut the dribble off at the pass.

Likely a combination of time and application, the intermittent stress incontinence I experienced postpartum with post-urination, sneezing, *spaztastic* laughing, and running has been remedied.

"A dribble." The universe was making sure I had not forgotten its magnificence, once again.

A dribble is how I entered labor and birth, my waters dribbling before my first birth started. A dribble is how I exited labor and birth, dribbling after my second.

"Nothing is ever going be the same," said my dear and delectable friend.

I look in the mirror these days, and I barely recognize what I see.

A smidge of that variation stems from what I believe is deeper nutrition promoting a healthy inside that does not necessarily provide my outside with the fleshiness I prefer, particularly in the derrière. The bubs could use a new suspension. The abs, where do I start? They feel a bit like a trampoline around the belly button. A belly button that is permanently "popped" in its own right. On their lower recesses, those abs model a scar that mimics a famous lopsided Hollywood smile. And the skin on them resembles that of a Shar-Pei's, which is nothing to scoff at. Quite symbolic and even encouraging, the Shar-Pei's loose skin actually served as body armor when originally bred by the ancient Chinese to guard the royal palace and protect the royal family.

I can see neither my work-in-progress pelvic floor nor my vagina that barely tore…but I know they are there. And I know what they did.

I know what this body did.

So I smile and I look straight into that mirror and I think you may not be what you used to be, but you are so much more. You fierce birthing body.

Remember the nursery rhyme, the cumulative tale *This Is the House That Jack Built*? I and my body consider ourselves privileged, as well as one-shot fledgling poets, to have a cumulative postpartum tale of our own.

Ahem...

*This Is the Body That Birth Built*

This is the taut skin and the perky bubs and the leg
That belonged to the runner showing no age
That met a man among men and got engaged
That fertilized what the runner laid
That nestled in a uterus and made some babes
That created a scar and a tear and fried eggs
That nourish and bond and flow like tapped kegs
That aren't the only things that drip and are worn
That challenge the core and the pelvic floor
That lay in the fierce body that birth built.

# He's Home

ELEVEN HOURS LATER:

Warm.

Intimate.

Homey.

"Hair. It's a head."

"Oh my gosh, babe, I can see it!"

"I can see a head."

"Oh my gosh, it's happening!"

"We're really doing this."

Wade, who said he did not want to see anything "down there," is peeking around my knee looking directly down there. I imagine his voice has not steeped in this timbre since he was a child on Christmas morning. It is delightful, really, witnessing in such a large man a glimpse of the little boy I never knew.

And I will never forget the look on his face—the excitement, the wonder—priceless and worth every push.

There are a few more...pushes. Before our child releases from my body the way a roasting hen does from its packaging. Decidedly what birthing a body reminds me of—slippery and wobbly, resistant at first, and then right on out.

Immediately, any pain is gone. It is glorious, a gargantuan relief. Knowing that baby is here and the hardest part is behind us, that simply and frankly the contractions are not coming back.

This is the everlasting part. The part that makes every other part worth doing. I understand why so many women share a common theme in their birth stories: the reward outweighs the work, the pain. Coming through something so challenging and quite possibly the most intensely acute physical, psychological event many may ever face is gratifying, empowering, amazing. Mother, baby, and birth partner facing it together, birth is life in microcosm. It is the unveiling of capacity in the face of adversity. It is the learning of lessons that are difficult to teach. It is a moment in time removed from the minutiae of life where one can witness how truly beautiful and extraordinary life is.

Even "extraordinary" is an understatement.

I can see it in Wade's expression and feel it in my own.

His hands do not know what to do. They cover his mouth then rake over his pooling eyes then thump over his racing heart, as electrified as the bounding chest in which it is encased. His eyes, as animated, dart back and forth from me to seconds-born babe.

"Ba-a-abe…" he whispers, full kissable bottom lip giving way to a quiver.

"I know…" I whisper back.

Momentarily stunned, I can't even cry. I thought I would. Or maybe I thought I should. Another birth pipe dream. I am just staring at this unfamiliar little face, not quite what I imagined but enchanting all the same.

"Hi, baby," I coo. Did we really just have you? My afterthought coos, too.

Baby gazes at me, equally astonished. In mere seconds his environment, world, life looks and feels different, distinct, strange. One thing he recognizes is my voice. He clings to it, eyes focused on nothing but me and widening with certain inflections of my tone.

While I make introductions, telling baby—who rests on my lower abdomen until the placenta is birthed and can follow him around—how happy we are to finally meet him, I think to myself, that's a boy, right? He just looks like a boy, whatever that connotes. If he is a girl, well then, she is the most handsome little thing I have ever seen!

Wade must muse over the same thing because he finally finds his voice. "Well, whatcha got down there?" he says to Genevieve and Katie and Erica, who discreetly tend to and monitor baby and me, allowing us to have our first-ever-laid-eyes-on-you moment free of intrusion.

"I don't know. You tell me. Come see for yourself," I paraphrase the tripled response, accompanied with smiles and shrugs.

I had told Genevieve we wanted to be surprised. We did, however, opt for a noninvasive genetic/chromosome blood test. Despite leaving the "gender reveal" box unchecked, the test revealed it anyhow in the form of an X or Y chromosome. Therefore, in checking and reporting results back to us, she was exposed to the gender. Although it would have been ideal for all of us to be surprised, she did a great job in not spilling the beans.

Once I knew that she knew, I thought it might be hard to refrain from knowing, but it wasn't. A few times Wade considered calling her to find out for himself, conflicted as to whether he wanted more the surprise or "preparation," he said. "Resolution," I said, knowing he hoped for a boy, seeing how we already had our girl.

"Here's Genevieve's number," I passed it to him on a Post-it note, "but don't you dare let it slip." I was fully committed to the surprise. Unusual in and of itself, considering I feel about surprises the way I feel about horror movies.

"I almost called Genevieve today," he must have said tens of times. Leaving me to consider, did he subconsciously crave the surprise or did he fear he could not keep the secret!

In all honesty, once I did try to read Genevieve by reading between the lines when we were talking casually about names.

"We like Maxim 'Max' Julius for a boy, after his Pawpaw Julius."

"Ahhh, what a strong name," she said with kind approval.

Strong? Is she saying there is a *strong* possibility we are expecting a boy? "And for a girl, we like Arena Pearl, after both great-grandmothers."

"Oooh, 'Arena Pearl,'" she repeated, all warm and inspired, possibly liking it even better than Maxim Julius, before adding, "what a unique name."

A girl, then! Or is she too impressed with the name? Leading me to think it's a girl when it's really a boy. If you really want to know, ask! The ol' nag summed it up for me. Apparently I didn't want to know, because I didn't...ask.

I am thankful I did not, translating to I am thankful I was patient. I am thankful Wade did not. I am thankful that the wise and thoughtful women attending us let him find out for himself, refraining from blurting out "It's a..."

The stupefaction or the triumph in Wade's expression as he looks for himself, I cannot say which thrills me more. He got his boy? He answers his own wonder with one firm handclap and a moderated "Yes!" His composure answering my question, he would have been just as grateful if *he* were another *she*.

Elation quickly turning to concern, "Why isn't he crying?" Wade asks, maybe now that he has a mind to.

Momentarily, I wonder the same thing, recalling Mila's worrisome question "Will Julian cry?"

But all I have to do is look at him. He is warm. He is pink. He has good muscle tone. His plump seraphic little figure, lying skin to skin against my abdomen, rises and falls relaxed of breath. His slate gray newborn eyes keep mine. They mesmerize and radiate with their own distinct brand of communication, more than words could ever say. He is neither a quiet soul nor an old one, as his serene hello to the world may suggest. He is a throwback, born on his great-uncle's eighty-third birthday. He has a confidence about himself, an easy freedom, an open-eyed awareness. He is taking it all in.

That is when my eyes flicker with moisture. We did it, baby boy. Just like we imagined in the sky blue birthing hammock—calm, trust, freedom.

"Is he okay? What's that sound?" Wade continues. To this day, I still do not know what sound he was talking about. "Is he having trouble breathing? Shouldn't he be crying?"

"He couldn't be any more perfect," Genevieve assuages. "Not all babies cry at birth." She shrugs with a keen smile. "Maybe he just knows..."

And she lets us fill in the blank...he's home.

# Placenta Party

GENEVIEVE WAS RIGHT. HE KNEW.

Attached to that bed as much as he is to Wade's and my chest, he will not entertain sleeping anywhere but one of the three. After nursing, rocking or walking him to sleep, we lay him in the bed he was made and born, and his mouth inevitably pulls up at the corners—a contented smile.

He's home.

Finally convinced his boy is okay, Wade ushers his best girl and firstborn into the bedroom.

From my vantage point, reclined and awaiting the placenta's arrival, I hear her before I see her sweet little mop of blonde hair making its way around the bed.

"Mama? Mama? I heard you making those noises. 'Grrrhhh...'" she impersonates, much like her daddy. "I wanted to come help you. Did you puuush that baby out?" She finally reaches me, Daddy helping her up onto the bed.

"I missed you!" I say, realizing I haven't been so long without her in I couldn't tell you when. "Yes...we did...puuush that baby out." A feat by which I am still stunned, as evidenced by the self-checking pauses. I reach an arm out to her.

What a feeling. One arm holding our newborn and one arm holding our firstborn. I had never felt split, torn, before as a mother. Which way? Which one? I have enough arms, energy, love for both, right? Somewhere in the thankfulness—double the love and joy, rounding out the family, how did we come/what did we do to ever deserve all of this—lurks uncertainty. How is it, exactly, we are to manage all of this? How do we give them both what they need without taking away from one or the other?

And I get my first tutorial, and heaping helping of guilt, as a new mother of two.

"Hahhh!" Mila inhales the surprise, laying eyes on Brother for the first time. I see the million questions, but she goes straight to a familiar and preliminary one with her elephant memory, "Did Julian cry? Why isn't he crying?"

I chuckle, thinking that even if she and her daddy were not look-alikes, no one would ever have to wonder were they flesh and blood. For their identical idiosyncrasies—which seems an oxymoron in itself—would give them away.

"Of course he didn't cry, not with you for a Big Sis," I say. "And we'll call him Max from now on. But we kept part of your *Julian*. His middle name is *Julius*. Maxim Julius. Max."

"Mmm-ax, like Mmm-ila," she accentuates recently studied phonetics.

"Yes, very good," I say to her. "And you did very good, too, son," I say to him, practicing this whole splitting the difference in attention thing.

"Max-a-mookah," she adds her own spin, which has stuck, determined to take part in the naming. "Why is he just lying there? Staring?"

I chuckle again, guessing in her busy toddler world that would be pretty boring. "You used to just lie there and stare, too. Those were some of my favorite times. Talking with you without saying a word. He'll get more exciting, I promise. Oh, no, honey, you can't touch his eyes." I intercept a curious hand before it reaches those "staring" eyes. Always with the eyes—stuffed animals, dolls, toys, anything with an eye—she wants to inspect. Future optometrist?

"Look what Brother brought you," Daddy says, introducing the oversized wrapped gift Grandma Glory delivers with impeccable timing.

The opposite of a parting gift, Big Buck is a greeting gift, a get-on-your-good-side-out-of-the-gate gift.

It works smashingly. Big Buck is the coolest thing since Minnie

Mouse. And Brother is even cooler for delivering him to her at his delivery, even if he is "boring."

Ooh, oh, ouch…a contraction? Please, for the love of all things painless, I thought we were done with those.

"Just a few more, bear down gently with them, if you want to," Genevieve mentors, intuitively reading my body language.

Ooh, oh, yeah…placenta! I was not expecting that, more contractions. Mild contracting, a pinch, maybe cramping, but not actual contractions. I guess I assumed that after baby paved the way it would just kind of wiggle on out. And it did…wiggle on out…after a few more contractions. A bit of a rude awakening in light of fifteen minutes without them after all day with them, even the few it took to birth the placenta seemed a few too many.

Although, the patience with which the placenta was birthed and treated swiftly countervailed the additional discomfort. There was no hurry, no manual maneuvering, no "external uterine massage" and/or "traction" on the exposed part of the umbilical cord, impatiently coaxing the placenta from a uterus that had labored all day and maybe just needed to catch its breath for a spell. There was no tossing of the birthed placenta into a biohazard waste bucket. The theme of my prenatal period played out in my immediate postpartum period, as the placenta too was used to educate.

After inspecting for herself that it was there in its entirety—that nothing got left behind in my uterus—Genevieve proceeded to teach me a bit about the self-contained organ that sustained a thirty-eight-week-and-six-day pregnancy. I shall forever treasure her sitting by my side in the bed Max was born while he breastfed for the very first time. Placenta in hand, she explained what had been attached to where and the functions of those parts. I loved it, giving time and attention to the selfless workhorse of my pregnancy, honoring it somehow. To be fully honored at a later date as the root of a birth tree, once we settle on a location and species of tree.

Mila even got in on the placenta party. After the cord stopped pulsating, and after she was assured it would not hurt Brother, she and

Daddy cut the cord in the space between where Genevieve clamped it, separating our boy from the charitable placenta and the utero world indefinitely.

The symbolism was most fitting. Likely a first of many instances, and in many ways, where Big Sis will cut Brother loose.

# Birthing Among Women

AFTER AN UNDISTURBED FIRST HOUR OF LIFE—NO SEPARATION OF MOTHER AND child—Wade got some highly anticipated bare-chested skin-to-skin bonding time with his newborn son, while I got a stitching up.

My first-degree perineal laceration would heal itself if I would adhere to bed rest and little activity for a week or so. With an active toddler in my midst, I opted for sutures instead.

In pre-home birth musings about home birth, I never could have imagined looking back on any stitching up as a highlight, much less as impressing. But it was. It did…impress upon me the virtue of birthing among women.

Marinating in post-birth euphoria, I was a regular Chatty Cathy. Genevieve, Katie, and Erica willingly entertained me, likely riding a bit of a successful birth high themselves.

What I came through with these women, what these women nurtured in me, I will always think of them with admiration and adoration. Acquaintances just nine months ago, in my birth they were sisters. Mothers, daughters, wives, women, the epitome of and literal translation of "midwife"—"with woman"—I am so fortunate they were with me.

Somewhere between that first undisturbed hour of life and my first postpartum shower, Genevieve, Katie, and Erica worked behind the scenes, much like they did throughout my labor and birth.

There was no chaos, no rounding up and marching in and out of staff and caregivers, no mass of beeps and alerts and machinery sounding off, no intrusion, no distress. Yet everyone who needed to be assessed, and everything that needed to be done, was. Even voluntary things, special and thoughtful touches, were complete.

Happy Mama Herbals postpartum sitz bath was steeped and ladled into peri bottles and over sanitary pads that would serve as relieving and healing perineal washes and ice packs. Considerately prepared in bulk, they were stored in my refrigerator and freezer for convenient use. Cleanup of the general area ensued, to include several trips in and out with suitcases full of birthing and postpartum and emergency supplies, not to mention the cumbersome disassembly and hauling off of the birthing tub. Sheets, towels, bedding, clothing, anything succumbed to laboring and birthing fluids was gathered up, washed, dried, and folded...for me, for us.

Talk about a pampering, feeling special in a community of women.

Once the i's got their dots and the t's their crosses, it must have been midnight. And what a relief to be home.

It is a cool November night. My go-to robe—vibrant red and adorned with hearts—a Valentine's gift from Mom, feels particularly plush wrapped around this fierce birthing body. The color is even appropriate. Red is the color of extremes. Red is the color of fire and blood, energy and primal life forces. I am quite certain I just experienced them all.

Albeit, I do not feel energetic in my red robe. My body found its ceiling under the massaging tempo of hot, steamy water. It seeks hibernation.

Genevieve escorts me to bed and tucks me in. Yes, she tucks me in, the way a mother would, the way a midwife does. She beckons our boy from the stingy clutches of his daddy. Their bond is complete. Both having enjoyed the therapeutic skin-to-skin session, they are peacefully heavy-eyed and blood-heavy with the "feel good," "cuddle hormone," natural "love drug" oxytocin.

I feel it, too, as soon as Genevieve hands him to me. An indescribable it—holding a newborn, our newborn. We have felt it before. Discovering it with a firstborn had to carry some weight in this very moment, the desire to feel it again with a second born. Likely our last hurrah, I mindfully cling to it.

I adore that this is how our home birth draws to a close. Genevieve accepts Max from Wade and gives him to me, tucking him to my skin beneath my robe. In the chain—Wade, Genevieve, me—Genevieve is the link. The one who believed in us. The one who believed in me and home birth when Wade was uncertain. The link that provided us an entirely new and fascinating bond in coming through a home birth together.

Fulfilling the romantic image I carry of early midwives answering and departing "the call"—riding out on bikes, buggies, even horseback like those I read about in the Appalachian Mountains—in the wee hours, Genevieve, Katie, and Erica retire from us.

Their *horses* of the four-wheeled persuasion and like most who have actually *sat in the saddle*, they probably would not classify their unusual and long hours as "romantic" but evocative, nonetheless.

When Genevieve leaves, I feel a rush of apprehension. What will we do without her? Then I recall those seven words she told me mere weeks after our initial meeting and as I was miscarrying: *Your body knows how to do this.*

Yes, it does. Yes, I do.

That miscarriage finally coming full circle, I exhale a mounting lump from the back of my throat. I am too tired to cry. I am too relieved to cry. I am too fortunate to cry.

"We are so thankful you are here," I whisper to the eight-pound cherub whose eyes give in to sleep. Who purrs like a bear cub against my chest.

Aside from gender, I discover the first apparent difference in my children. Mila was not so much a purrer but a grunter, a melodic one, of course!

And here she comes *riding* Big Buck. "Mama, may I sleep with Grandma Glory tonight?"

I don't know why she asks. I figured she would, seeing how we are old hat when Grandma comes to town. "Sure, baby," I whisper. Everything at this point is a whisper, the moo-howl-roar having fatigued my vocal cords.

"What's that sound?"

"That's Brother, love."

"What's wrong with him?"

Oh, Lord, not this again. "You and your daddy, child." I chuckle with amusement and fondness and slight exasperation at their likeness. "Nothing is wrong with him. He's just so happy to be with us, he's purring…you know, like a kitty purrs when you pet it."

"And I'm so happy he brought me this Big Buck. Maybe you could push another baby out and I could get another Big Buck?"

Baaahahahahaaa!

# Notes

*Birthing From Within* emerged as a consistent source throughout this memoir, specifically in chapters Chant Sheet, Pain Cube, and The Lizard & The Lotus, considering the book was the bedrock of my preparation for labor and birth. Warmly referred to as *BFW* with subsequent mentions, the abbreviation is to me an endearment. For the book is to me a familiar friend.

Pam England & Rob Horowitz, *Birthing From Within*, Partera Press, 1998.

Any book pertaining to birth would not be complete without the inspiration and readings of Ina May Gaskin. Her insights and quotes are speckled throughout this memoir like accenting strokes a painter leaves on canvas, only making it deeper and more intriguing to the eye. It was through Ina May's writings that I first understood all that is and can be birth.

Ina May Gaskin, *Birth Matters: A Midwife's Manifesta*, Seven Stories Press, 2011.

Ina May Gaskin, *Ina May's Guide to Breastfeeding: From the Nation's Leading Midwife*, Bantam, 2009.

Ina May Gaskin, *Ina May's Guide to Childbirth*, Bantam Dell, 2003.

Ina May Gaskin, *Spiritual Midwifery*, Book Publishing Company, 2002.

Part I

I Know Nothing

1. "Our Brains Control Our Thoughts, Feelings, and Behaviors," *Introduction to Psychology*, University of Minnesota, 2015, http://open.lib.umn.edu/intropsyc/chapter/3-2-our-brains-control-our-thoughts-feelings-and-behavior/.

Nurse Curse

1. World Health Organization, "WHO Statement on Caeserean Section Rates," Switzerland: World Health Organization, 2015, http://apps.who.int/iris/bitstream/10665/161442/1/WHO_RHR_15.02_eng.pdf.

Come Undone

1. Katherine Hartmann and others, "Outcomes of Routine Episiotomy A Systematic Review," *JAMA*, 2005;293(17):2141–2148, https://jamanetwork.com/journals/jama/fullarticle/200799.

Dumb Luck

1. Charles Newlin and others, "Cesarean Section Incision Complications and Associated Risk Factors: A Quality Assurance Project," *Open Journal of Obstetrics and Gynecology*, 2015, 5, 789-794, http://file.scirp.org/pdf/OJOG_2015113015463561.pdf.

2. The American Congress of Obstetricians and Gynecologists, "ACOG Releases New Guidance Aimed at Making VBAC Available to More Women," ACOG, 2017, www.acog.org/About-ACOG/News-Room/News-Releases/2017/ACOG-Releases-New-Guidance-Aimed-at-Making-VBAC-Available-to-More-Women.

More Is Less

1. Robbie E. Davis-Floyd, *Birth as an American Rite of Passage*, University of California Press, 2004.

2. Carol Peckham, "Medscape Malpractice Report 2015: Why Ob/Gyns Get Sued," *Medscape*, WebMD, 2016, https://www.medscape.com/features/slideshow/malpractice-report-2015/obgyn.

3. Nell Lake, "Labor, Interrupted—Cesareans, 'cascading interventions,' and finding a sense of balance," *Harvard Magazine*, November-December 2012, www.harvardmagazine.com/2012/11/labor-interrupted.

Insufficient Knowledge

1. "Cervidil: Important Safety Information," Ferring Pharmaceuticals, 2015, www.cervidil.com/hcp/important-safety-information/.

2. E Lieberman and others, "Changes in fetal position during labor and their association with epidural analgesia," *Obstet Gynecol.*, 2005;105:974–982, www.ncbi.nlm.nih.gov/pubmed/15863533.

The Average Woman

1. Rebecca Dekker, "Evidence on: Premature Rupture of Membranes," *Evidenced Based Birth*, 2017, https://evidencebasedbirth.com/evidence-inducing-labor-water-breaks-term/.

What More

1. Megan McArdle, "Life Without Antibiotics Would Be Nasty, Brutish and Short(er): The rise of antibiotic resistance is one of the world's greatest health challenges," *Bloomberg.com*, 2013, www.bloomberg.com/view/articles/2013-09-18/life-without-antibiotics-would-be-nasty-brutish-and-short-er-.

2. M.P. Francino, "Antibiotics and the Human Gut Microbiome: Dysbioses and Accumulation of Resistances," *Frontiers in Microbiology*, 6 (2015): 1543, www.ncbi.nlm.nih.gov/pmc/articles/PMC4709861/.

Just In Case

1.  Abhishek Deshpande and others, "Antibiotic-Associated Diarrhea and *Clostridium Difficile.*" Cleveland Clinic Center for Continuing Education, 2014, https://teachmemedicine.org/cleveland-clinic-antibiotic-associated-diarrhea-and-clostridium-difficile/.

2.  Susanne Hempel and others, "Probiotics for the Prevention and Treatment of Antibiotic-Associated Diarrhea," *JAMA*, 2012;307(18):1959-1669, https://pdfs.semanticscholar.org/7dc7/b4872250e6defa8f4be1a7f8594dca3281fd.pdf.

3.  Martin H. Floch, "Recommendations for Probiotic Use in Humans—A 2014 Update," *Pharmaceuticals*, 2014, 7, 999-1007, http://www.mdpi.com/1424-8247/7/10/999/htm.

4.  Jon A. Vanderhoof and Rosemary Young, "Probiotics in the United States," *Clinical Infectious Diseases*, Volume 46, Issue Supplement_2, 1 February 2008, Pages S67–S72, https://doi.org/10.1086/523339.

Slow Learner

1.  Jennifer A. Unger and others, "The Emergence of *Clostridium difficile* Infection among Peripartum Women: A Case-Control Study of a *C. difficile* Outbreak on an Obstetrical Service," *Infectious Diseases in Obstetrics and Gynecology*, vol. 2011, Article ID 267249, 8 pages, 2011, https://doi.org/10.1155/2011/267249.


Part II

Tripartite

1.  M. Lemmers and others, "Dilatation and curettage increases the risk of subsequent preterm birth: a systematic review and meta-analysis," *Human Reproduction*, Volume 31, Issue 1, 1 January 2016, Pages 34–45, https://doi.org/10.1093/humrep/dev274.

2.  Charles Butler and others, "How long is expectant management safe in first-trimester miscarriage?," *J Fam Pract.*, 2005 October;54(10):889-890, https://www.mdedge.com/jfponline/article/61032/womens-health/how-long-expectant-management-safe-first-trimester-miscarriage.

Chant Sheet

1.  Eric Jensen, *Teaching with the Brain in Mind*, Association for Supervision and Curriculum Development, 2005, www.ascd.org/publications/books/104013/chapters/Movement-and-Learning.aspx.

Data...Yawn

1.  Melissa Cheyney and others, "Outcomes of Care for 16,924 Planned Home Births in the United States: The Midwives Alliance of North America Statistics

Project, 2004 to 2009," *Journal of Midwifery & Women's Health*, 59: 17–27, 2014, http://onlinelibrary.wiley.com/doi/10.1111/jmwh.12172/epdf.

2. Manchester University, "Natural births after caesarean more likely if you call the midwife," *ScienceDaily*, 20 April 2016, www.sciencedaily.com/releases/2016/04/160420090056.htm.

Nurses On Horseback

1. Najla Barnawi and others, "Midwifery and Midwives: A Historical Analysis," *J. Res. Nurs. Midwifery* 2(8):114-121, 2013, https://www.interesjournals.org/articles/midwifery-and-midwives-a-historical-analysis.pdf.

2. Adrian E. Feldhusen, "The History of Midwifery and Childbirth in America: A Time Line," *Midwifery Today*, 2000, www.midwiferycollege.org/AcademicProgram/Downloads/ASM/Academics/Syllabi/historyofmidwifery/History%20of%20Midwifery%20-%20Midwifery%20TodayPdf.pdf.

3. Abraham Flexner and Daniel B. Updike, *Medical Education in the United States and Canada: A Report to the Carnegie Foundation for the Advancement of Teaching*, publisher not identified, 1910, www.credentialwatch.org/reports/flexner_1910.pdf.

4. Judith Walzer Leavitt, "Joseph B. DeLee and the Practice of Preventive Obstetrics," *AJPH*, October 1988, Vol. 78, No 10 page 1353, www.ncbi.nlm.nih.gov/pmc/articles/PMC1349440/pdf/amjph00249-0095.pdf.

5. "History of FNU," Frontier Nursing University, https://frontier.edu/about-frontier/history-of-fnu/.

6. Mary Breckinridge, *Wide Neighborhoods: A Story of the Frontier Nursing Service*, University Press of Kentucky, 1981.

7. "Preliminary Report of 2,844 Pregnancies: 1970-2010," The Farm Midwifery Center, http://thefarmmidwives.org/preliminary-statistics/.

8. "There's a shortage of OB-GYNs and midwives. Here's what's being done about it," *Advisory.com*, The Advisory Board Company, September 1, 2016, www.advisory.com/daily-briefing/2016/09/01/ob-gyn-shortage.

9. Marian F. MacDorman and others, "Trends in Out-of-Hospital Births in the United States, 1990–2012," NCHS Data Brief, No. 144, March 2014, https://www.cdc.gov/nchs/data/databriefs/db144.htm.

Nesting

1. Gavin S Dawe and others, "Cell Migration from Baby to Mother," *Cell Adhesion & Migration*, 1.1 (2007): 19–27, www.ncbi.nlm.nih.gov/pmc/

articles/PMC2633676/.

2. "Red raspberry leaf," *ScienceDirect*, Elsevier, B.V., 2018, https://www.sciencedirect.com/topics/medicine-and-dentistry/red-raspberry-leaf.

3. Happy Mama Herbals Postpartum Sitz Bath, *Texas Medicinals*, Ginger Webb, 2018, https://gingerwebb.com/texas-medicinals/herbs-for-mamas/sitz-bath/.

4. American Society For Microbiology, "Birds Use Herbs To Protect Their Nests," *ScienceDaily*, 27 May 2004, www.sciencedaily.com/releases/2004/05/040527080935.htm.

Part III

Adventure Of A Lifetime

1. Sarah Clark, "Why I Love Transition Labor (And You Might Too)," *Mama Birth*, 2013, www.mamabirth.com/2013/08/why-i-love-transition-labor-and-you.html.

The Body That Birth Built

1. Nicole Crawford, "Stop Doing Kegels: Real Pelvic Floor Advice For Women (And Men)," *BreakingMuscle.com*, http://breakingmuscle.com/fitness/stop-doing-kegels-real-pelvic-floor-advice-for-women-and-men.

2. Kelly I. Daly and Jennifer Doherty-Restrepo, "Stress Urinary Incontinence in Female Athletes," Florida International University, https://pdfs.semanticscholar.org/30e6/4a1f89d52b797a7b52df041752c4d243d810.pdf.

3. "Physiotherapy Works: The Evidence—Urinary Incontinence," Physiotherapy New Zealand, 2018, https://physiotherapy.org.nz/assets/95f9c52b9d/PNZ-Urinary-Incontinence-v2.pdf.

4. Katy Bowman, "You (Still) Don't Know Squat," *Nutritious Movement*, 2013, https://nutritiousmovement.com/you-still-dont-know-squat/.

5. Alanna Ketler, "The Forgotten Art Of Squatting: Is It The Antidote For The Damage Done To Our Bodies From Sitting?," *Collective Evolution*, 2018, https://www.collective-evolution.com/2018/02/22/the-forgotten-art-of-squatting-is-it-the-antidote-for-the-damage-done-to-our-bodies-from-sitting/.

# Gratitude

Wade, Mila, and Maxim, how will I ever thank you for showing me a life I never dreamed of that is more than anything I ever wanted. I love the bones of you. "Just one more chapter," I must have said a hundred times before escaping to the back bedroom. Beautiful man, your selfless double daddy duty only further stroked the fire down in my soul. Undoubtedly, it left its own impression on the souls of our children. Beautiful children, your fair understanding and commanding of my time made for the quintessential work-life harmony. The enthusiasm and inspiration the three of you provide make possible for me anything and everything.

Ma, it is staggering yet only appropriate how being a mother brings to one's attention how much their own mother has done and endured and tried. For it all, I adore you.

Ange and Nett—sisters, mothers, confidants, my Wonder Women—I am better for your mothering, too.

Gram, you made loving and mothering and home-birthing children through The Great Depression seem like a walk in the park. The coolest, grittiest, wittiest, near-centenarian matriarch I ever knew, what a legacy you left us.

Oma, Memaw, Grandma Glory, Nana, and Gamaw—great-grandmothers, grandmothers, and mothers—our children are so very fortunate to have you. Keepers of family and powerful influencers, not only are we born through you, the way those born through us see themselves is enriched by your complete love.

Genevieve Schaefer—midwife, mother, birth sage—you are thought of often with awe-inspiring warmth and gratitude. Forever a part of our birth love story, thank you for the adventure of a lifetime.

Miriam McKinney—childbirth educator, mother—your sincere candor and constructive insights on a very rough draft were much needed and sincerely appreciated. Your talents cease to amaze me.

Rachel McCarty—registered nurse, mother—your comprehensive notes and well-rounded acumen on my first pass greatly improved all of my other passes. You rock.

Cynthia Gage—editor, exquisite mother to an exquisite son—through whom the potential of this memoir in its finest form was actualized. I give you my heartfelt thanks for your expert safekeeping and hard work. For encouraging and empowering me. For lifting up what I do by doing what you do so well. For showing me that birthing and writing have much in common. That as I came to learn to trust in, surrender to, and accept the natural process of birth, I came to learn to trust in, surrender to, and accept the natural process of editing. It has made all the difference. With love and appreciation, thank you, thank you, thank you.

Birth, what haven't you taught me? In the debate concerning how you are to be done, let us not forget the rite and the right. Surely we can all come together in solidarity for choice, support of choice, ultimately healthy and happy mothers and babies.

# About The Author

Brooklyn James is an author/singer-songwriter inspired by life in the *Live Music Capital* of Austin, Texas. Her first novel, *The Boots My Mother Gave Me,* has an original music soundtrack and was chosen as a Quarter Finalist in the Amazon Breakthrough Novel Awards. The book provided a platform where it was her honor to serve as a guest speaker with a focus on awareness and prevention of domestic violence and suicide.

When she is not writing books, she can be found playing live music around Austin as part of an acoustic duo. Moonlighting occasionally in voice-over and film, she played a Paramedic in a Weezer video, met Harry Connick Jr. as an extra on the set of *When Angels Sing,* appeared in Richard Linklater's *Boyhood* for all of a nanosecond, and was a stand-in and stunt double for Mira Sorvino on Jerry Bruckheimer's *Trooper* pilot for TNT. Although reading, dancing, working out, and a good glass of kombucha get her pretty excited, she finds most thrilling the privilege of being a mother to two illuminating little souls and a wife to the one big soul from whom they get their light.

Brooklyn holds an M.A. in Communication, and a B.S. in both Nursing and Animal Science. Her nursing career has seen specialties in the areas of Intensive Care and Postpartum. With the publication of her birth memoir, she is available for speaking engagements, readings, signings, and writing workshops on how to put pen to paper composing one's own birth story.

She thanks you kindly for your time and reading attention, and she would be delighted if you may consider leaving a review for *Born in the Bed You Were Made.*

Find her at brooklyn-james.com or facebook.com/BrooklynJamesAuthor.

Made in the USA
Lexington, KY
09 September 2019